Nursing Assessment, Plan of Care, and Patient Education

The Foundation of Patient Care

Pamela Craig, RN, BSN

Patricia R. Dolan, RN, BSN, MSN

Kevin Drew, RNC

Patricia Pejakovich, RN, BSN, MPA, CPHQ

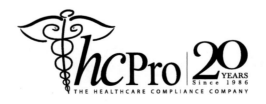

Nursing Assessment, Plan of Care, and Patient Education: The Foundation of Patient Care is published by HCPro, Inc.

Copyright 2006 HCPro, Inc.

ISBN 1-57839-798-7

HCPro, Inc., provides information resources for the healthcare industry.

HCPro, Inc., is not affiliated in any way with the Joint Commission on Accreditation of Healthcare Organizations, which owns the JCAHO trademark.

Pamela Craig, RN, BSN, Author
Patricia Dolan, RN, BSN, MSN, Author
Kevin Drew, RNC, Author
Patricia Pejakovich, RN, BSN, MPA, CPHQ, Author
John Novack, Group Publisher
Molly Hall, Executive Editor

Amy Anthony, Senior Managing Editor
Jean St. Pierre, Director of Operations
Shane Katz, Cover Designer
Jackie Diehl Singer, Graphic Artist
Crystal Beland, Layout Artist

Advice given is general. Readers should consult professional counsel for specific legal, ethical, or clinical questions.

Arrangements can be made for quantity discounts. For more information, contact:

HCPro, Inc.
P.O. Box 1168
Marblehead, MA 01945
Telephone: 800/650-6787 or 781/639-1872
Fax: 781/639-2982
E-mail: *customerservice@hcpro.com*

103.20   616.075
Nur

Visit HCPro at its World Wide Web site:
www.hcpro.com

CONTENTS

ABOUT THE AUTHORS

Pamela Craig, RN, BSN

Pamela Craig, RN, BSN is the chief nursing officer at Brownwood Regional Medical Center in Brownwood, TX, a member of the Triad Hospital Corporation. She specializes in analysis and development of nursing systems, with a special focus on integration of the nursing process at all levels of service, including administration.

Pamela has been devoted to nursing for more than 21 years, beginning as a staff nurse in various clinical settings, including medical/surgical, psychiatry, and women's services. Early in her career, she developed an interest in the efficient organization of nursing services, with an emphasis on both patient outcome and nursing satisfaction. Her interest and skills in these areas were further developed in a community health center setting where she worked as a health educator and eventually advanced to become assistant director. She has been with Brownwood Regional Medical Center for the past six years, starting as nursing projects director, and three years ago advanced to her current position of chief nursing officer.

Pamela's approach to the organization of nursing services stems from a true love of the art of nursing and nurses themselves, as well as a long-standing interest in creating efficient methods for providing services. Her philosophy of leadership is based on an investment in staff ownership of nursing processes and her belief that nursing services cannot be provided at the expense of nurses. She uses the nursing process itself as a means of analyzing the component parts of services—which she compares to interacting puzzle pieces—with patient outcomes and employee satisfaction being of equal importance. In her leadership role, she focuses on the interrelationship of staff, patients, and management, and her leadership hallmark is the ability to develop and analyze systems while coaching and developing leadership among her staff.

Pamela received her bachelor of science in nursing from Grand Canyon College (now Grand Canyon University) in Phoenix, AZ. She is a member of the American Organization of Nurse Executives, the Texas Organization of Nurse Executives, and the Texas Nurses Association.

Patricia R. Dolan, RN, BSN, MSN

Patricia R. Dolan, RN, BSN, MSN is currently the chief nursing officer for Saint Mary's Regional Medical Center in Russellville, AK. Patricia has served in clinical and administrative roles in large hospital systems, both not-for-profit, and for-profit for 30 years. She has successfully assisted hospitals in maintaining accreditation from the Joint Commission on Accreditation of Healthcare Organizations (JCAHO).

Patricia received both her master's degree in community health management and her bachelor's degree in nursing from the University of Memphis in Memphis, TN. She is a member of the American College of Health Care Executives, the American Organization of Nurse Executives, the Arkansas Organization of Nurse Executives, and Sigma Theta Tau.

Kevin Drew, RNC

Kevin Drew, RNC is the nurse manager of a 38-bed medical floor that cares for adult medical patients, pediatric patients, and oncology patients at McKenzie-Willamette Medical Center, a non-profit, 114-bed, acute-care facility in Springfield, OR.

In his 20 years in healthcare and 15 years in nursing, he has worked in various settings, including long-term care and medical/surgical, and has held both floor and administrative positions.

Kevin graduated from Lane Community College and Oregon Health Sciences University School of Nursing in Eugene, OR. He has worked at McKenzie-Willamette Medical Center since 1994. While at McKenzie-Willamette Medical Center, he has been instrumental in the complete reconstruction of the hospital's care-delivery system on the medical floor and has served on the hospital's Information Technology Steering Committee and the Patient Care Council.

Patricia Pejakovich, RN, BSN, MPA, CPHQ

Patricia Pejakovich, RN, BSN, MPA, CPHQ is a senior consultant for The Greeley Company, a division of HCPro, Inc., specializing in quality and performance improvement, accreditation, utilization management, credentialing, and data management and design. To assist clients in improving organizational operations, she brings 30 years of experience in nursing and healthcare, including more than 20 years of expertise in quality and performance improvement.

Prior to becoming a full-time consultant for The Greeley Company, Patricia served in administrative roles for hospitals, a health plan, and a healthcare consulting company. She has successfully led hospitals, health plans, credentialing verification organizations, and ambulatory facilities to achieve accreditation from JCAHO, the Healthcare Facilities Accreditation Program (HFAP) of the American Osteopathic Association, the National Committee for Quality Assurance (NCQA), and URAC, an independent accrediting organization. She has provided educational presentations to healthcare entities and professional organizations on such topics as credentialing, performance improvement, and quality management. Patricia has provided continuing medical educational programs for the Michigan State Medical Society on such subjects as utilization and quality management in a managed care environment.

Patricia's approach to integrating accreditation with organizational operations has resulted in accolades from her clients. She devises innovative and efficient methods to achieve improvement while decreasing or eliminating labor-intensive processes. Her ability to assess an organization's strengths and weaknesses, formulate an action plan, and motivate the participants to achieve successful outcomes, while adding a touch of humor, has been a key element of her clients' successes.

Patricia received her master's degree in public administration/healthcare at Western Michigan University in Kalamazoo, MI; and her bachelor's degree in nursing from the University of Michigan in Ann Arbor, Michigan she is also certified in healthcare quality (CPHQ). She is a member of the National Association for Healthcare Quality, the Michigan Association for Healthcare Quality, and Sigma Theta Tau.

INTRODUCTION

Assessment, care plans, and patient education

Over time, professional nursing has evolved from basic bedside tasks to critical, highly technical patient care. Models of nursing have emerged with the intent of providing higher quality of care with more efficiency. Regardless if nursing is practiced with a team approach or a primary care model, the discipline's foundation of care begins with a complete and accurate patient assessment. Data obtained from the assessment are then formulated into a plan of care, a dynamic document that is specific to the patient's needs. This plan of care is then intertwined with the education of both the patient and the patient's family. Without the implementation of these three functions, nursing care becomes reactive and is practiced as tasks in response to physician's orders.

As nurses, we have been educated to perform patient assessments and subsequently develop care plans utilizing critical thinking skills ingrained in us through rigorous course work and clinical experiences. The "educational model" of these documents was very much a regurgitation of all aspects of anatomy, physiology, basic nursing skills, pharmacology, and so on. Transitioning into the world of an extremely busy healthcare organization where a nurse's patient assignment far exceeds the student nurse's one or two patients may have resulted in a less-than-adequate performance of documented assessments and care plans. Nurses often become overloaded and focus on the tasks required of them, and complete the assessment and care plan as a paper form only and continue to "cognitively" process the patient's care.

So what did we do? We complicated matters by developing even more detailed and complex assessments and care plans, fitting in education as a component of the discharge instructions as we were rolling the patient out the door. We also began collecting far too much information than could be addressed during the drastically reduced lengths of hospital stays, and formulating pages and pages of canned care plans driven from one or several medical diagnoses. Nurses were drowning in worthless paper or electronic documents and yet, delivering highly complex care based on a thorough shift report. That well-used pocketed paper that directed the patient's care for the entire shift was indeed a nurse's assessment and care plan, but unfortunately it usually came to rest in the trash can.

The purpose of this book

Enough we say! Simplify, simplify, simplify is the message you will find in this book's pages. Whether your assessments, care plans, and education records are in hard copy or electronic versions, you will benefit from learning from experienced nurses about how to achieve success with these tools. They were developed by nurses for nurses and will be assets to the practice of nursing and not paper burdens like many current tools.

This book will provide you with realistic solutions to the chronic problems of documenting nursing practices in a time when nurses are in short supply and healthcare systems are expected to provide more with less. The authors' experiences will motivate you to assess your nursing practice and documentation methods.

The book's authors will provide you with detailed information on how they developed and implemented these essential nursing tools. They will share their experiences with you, both positive and negative, so you can determine what might be the most helpful steps for your organization to take to duplicate their successes. Copies of their tools are provided on a CD-ROM so you can customize them to your organization. If your facility has an electronic medical record, the fields within the vendor's documents could be edited to mirror the hardcopy version.

In my role as a consultant, I have had the pleasure of working with each of the authors. They are seasoned nursing leaders who share a passion for their profession and who work with their nursing staff to seek innovative solutions in eliminating barriers to efficient nursing practice. Interestingly, each of the authors works in hospitals separated by many miles but their facilities are very similar in size and services. Their hospitals are community based and not in large metropolitan areas, once again demonstrating that bigger is not always better.

Take the time to learn from them and jumpstart your nursing staff's desire to streamline required documentation, resulting in more time at the bedside. Your patients will thank you.

—Patricia Pejakovich, RN, BSN, MPA, CPHQ

Admission assessment

About this facility

Brownwood Regional Medical Center, Brownwood, TX

- 196 licensed beds
- Key services: ambulatory/outpatient, cardiology, emergency medicine ICU, oncology, orthopedics, physical/occupational medicine, radiology imaging, skilled nursing/rehab, surgical, women's and children's
- Last JCAHO survey: July 2005

Admission assessment

Introduction

The admission assessment is the fundamental baseline assessment which begins the nursing process of assessment, nursing diagnosis, planning, intervention, and evaluation. This assessment is a critical first step in the patient's care and serves as the first complete introduction the nurse has to the patient. During this process, the nurse assesses the patient from head to toe and establishes a baseline assessment. This baseline provides a point of reference for other nurses to compare against to see if the patient's condition is improving or declining. The admission assessment also points out problem areas to the nurse, which allows him or her to write a care plan that will guide the nursing staff in their care of the patient.

For example, a patient may be admitted with pneumonia, but during the assessment the nurse notes that the patient has experienced significant weight loss and is at risk for skin breakdown because she has poor skin turgor, and is immobile and incontinent. The nurse would write a care plan on the pneumonia as it relates to the patient's altered breathing status and appropriate nursing interventions. Additionally, the nurse could write a care plan on the patient's risk for skin breakdown and nursing interventions to reduce the patient's risk for developing a decubitus ulcer. The nurse could also make a referral to the dietitian to help with the patient's nutritional status.

In the spring of 2005, this important first step in a patient's care was found to be lacking in our facility, and we jumpstarted a collaborative effort of administration and staff nurses to revamp our admission assessment form.

The admission assessment form discussed in this chapter was developed through an administrative adaptation of the nursing process. The project began after the initial findings of a consultant we hired to help us prepare for our Joint Commission on Accreditation of Healthcare Organizations (JCAHO) survey. Her findings triggered an examination of the hospital staff's application of the nursing process, specifically as it applied to the development and updating of nursing care plans. When the problem with care plans was identified, a multilevel plan was developed which included input and reevaluation by administrative and direct-care staff. The project continued until the care-planning process was successfully improved. This chapter will walk you through the nursing process as it was applied to improving our admission assessment form.

Identifying the problem

In April of 2005, three months before the hospital's JCAHO survey, our facility's consultant noted that the staff's care planning was not thorough enough. The consultant observed that there was insufficient focus on priority issues and the care plans addressed more problems than could adequately be addressed. As a result, there was inadequate updating of the patient's care plan during his or her hospital stay. After much deliberation, which is detailed below, we learned it was our nursing assessment form that was leading to this poor care planning.

Assessment

In response to the consultant's assessment, I began to investigate the entire care-planning process: the initial assessment form, how it was used, what conclusion it rendered, and how the care plan itself was activated and reevaluated. At this initial phase, I informed the members of the nursing management team of the problem and interviewed them for their feedback concerning the care-planning process. This initial involvement of the team not only brought the problem to the forefront of the nurse managers' thinking, it also initiated their ownership for the development of a solution.

As the nursing management team brainstormed in this initial phase, they made several proposals, the strongest of which was revising the entire care plan to be standardized in care-path format. This seemed like a good idea, but the amount of time needed to accomplish this solution was not available because our survey was to take place in just three months. There also was not enough conclusive evidence that this would result in an efficient and effective solution. We needed to continue to investigate the problem, so I started to review the nursing process as it existed and as it applied to care plans. In this review, it became very clear that care planning depends upon the nursing process, and the nursing process is predicated upon the baseline nursing assessment. At this point, I suspected the problem was with the initial assessment process. This realization led to a full analysis of the nursing admission assessment process and care-plan development. To confirm this hunch, I examined the existing assessment forms and interviewed nurse managers regarding their experiences with the form. The nurse managers had utilized the existing form or some adaptation of the original for years. However, I had not, and this provided the advantage of a fresh perspective. This new perspective is something to consider when you are trying to analyze why your documentation is not getting the results you think it should. Invest in a review by other staff who do not currently utilize the document. It is amazing how another perspective can provide insight that those too close to the process cannot see.

The essential format of the existing baseline nursing assessment had been used for many years. Although the staff was quite familiar with its format, it contained several identifiable flaws. It had been typeset and printed internally. A hospital secretary completed the typesetting, and she was very accommodating and willing to "work in" modifications as requested. New JCAHO standards or practice updates were often inserted wherever they could be worked into the form. Because the form was often photocopied, it occasionally was crooked on the page and hard to read. Most importantly, I noted that it did not provide a summary section for the nurse to consolidate his or her findings in preparation for the care plan, nor did it provide a summary section for other care members to review. My overall impression was that the double-column format interfered with the flow of the assessment itself (see figure 1.1 for an example), the sequence of the assessment wasn't well organized or logical, and the form did not provide for a summary conclusion from which to develop a thorough care plan. Refer to figure 1.1 for an excerpt from this old assessment form. The excerpt is page one of the five-page form.

Diagnosis

I formulated a hypothesis based upon the above findings and my knowledge of the nursing process. My hypothesis was that the admission assessment was the key to satisfactory care planning and it was the process that required revision. I tested this theory by interviewing various members of the nursing management team. During these informal interviews, I learned that the nurses didn't necessarily like the form, but they had been using it for so long that they were uncertain about how to approach the process differently. They also pointed out that the form didn't follow a standard head-to-toe assessment, but rather it jumped around, in an inefficient manner. And, they said, the admis-

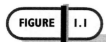

Previous patient admission assessment sheet

FIGURE 1.1

Check all that apply

Date: _____ **Time:** _____ O₂ Sat _____	**FAMILY HISTORY:** (List Whom) DISEASE OF:
T _____ P _____ R _____ B/P: RT _____ LT _____	☐ Heart _____
HT _____ **WT** _____ ☐ Upright ☐ Bed ☐ Stated	☐ D.M. _____
MODE: ☐ Ambulatory ☐ Stretcher ☐ Bed ☐ W/C	☐ Lung _____
ADMITTED FROM: ☐ ER ☐ MD Office ☐ Home ☐ NsgHm	☐ Cancer _____
ALLERGIES: _____	☐ Mind _____
_____	☐ Stroke _____
	☐ Other _____

LATEX ALLERGY SCREEN: Do you have: ☐ None

☐ Systemic symptoms from contact with balloons or gloves?
☐ A history of asthma?
Are you allergic to: ☐ bananas ☐ pineapple ☐ avocados
☐ A history of multiple urologic surgeries?
● *If you answer yes on 4 or more of the positive fields, notify physician of possible latex allergy.*

Signature: _____ **LVN/RN** _____

INFORMATION OBTAINED FROM: ☐ Patient ☐ Family
☐ S.O. ☐ Old Chart ☐ NsgHm Sheet ☐ Other
☐ Consent given to obtain information from family / S.O.

PT. CHIEF COMPLAINT/DURATION:

NUTRITIONAL ASSESSMENT:

Diet: _____
Food Intolerances: _____
☐ Weight change > 10 lb. within the last month
☐ Changes in appetite/intake > 3 days
☐ Nausea/Vomiting/Diarrhea > 3 days
☐ Decubitis ___ Stage II
☐ TPN/Tube Feed/PEG tube present
☐ Diagnosis of malnutrition, failure to thrive and/or Gestational Dia Mellitus.

CONSULT DIETICIAN IF ANY OF THE ABOVE ARE CHECKED.

WHO TO CALL IN AN EMERGENCY: _____

DO YOU HAVE: Power of Attorney for Health Care ☐ Y
If yes, _____
Name of Person with Power of Attorney/Relationship Telephone

DO YOU HAVE: Living Will ☐ Y ☐ N If **no** Living Will:
Was patient given additional literature? ☐ Y ☐ Patient D
Social Services Consult? ☐ Y ☐ N ☐ N/A

If patient **has** a Living Will, is
OR

HISTORY/PAST MEDICAL TX:
☐ Alcohol Use
☐ Cancer ☐ Heart ☐ Hypertension
☐ Diabetes ☐ Kidney ☐ Stroke
☐ Hepatitis ☐ Seizures ☐ Lung
☐ Ulcer ☐ Emotional/Psych
☐ Tobacco Use
☐ Smoking Cessation Education Provided
Other: _____

SURGERY: _____

Copy in Medical Records ☐ Ye:
Placed on chart ☐ Yes
Patient/Family to bring ☐ Ye:
Not Available ☐ Yes

If I, the patient, have a Living Will and a copy is not available, the substance of my advance directive is:

1) *DO NOT* prolong my life with life-sustaining treatment if I have a medical condition which can be reasonably expected to result in my imminent death.

2) If I am in a coma which my attending physician believes is irreversible, *DO NOT* prolong my life with life-sustaining treatment.

Flu Shot given within past 12-months? ☐ Yes ☐ No
Pneumonia Shot ☐ Yes (*Date Given* _____)
Offered: ☐ Accepted ☐ Declined

TB SCREENING: ☐ None Known
☐ Do you have, or have you ever had TB? Or do you have:
☐ Cough (>2wks) ☐ Night Sweats ☐ Bloody Sputum
☐ Fever ☐ Weight Loss ☐ Lack of Appetite
☐ None ☐ Previously Tested: ☐ Pos ☐ Neg

MEDS SENT: ☐ Home ☐ Pharmacy

3) I WANT MY LIFE TO BE PROLONGED TO THE GREATEST EXTENT POSSIBLE WITHOUT REGARD TO MY CONDITION, THE CHANCES I HAVE FOR RECOVERY, OR THE COST OF THE PROCEDURES.

Patient Signature _____ Date _____

Signature _____ RN Date/Time _____

Form #3370 (*REV 4-05*)

Place Patient Identification Sticker Here

Nursing Assessment, Plan of Care, and Patient Education: The Foundation of Patient Care

sion process was cumbersome, taking approximately 45 minutes per patient. After the interviews, it was clear to me that the nursing assessment form itself wasn't leading nurses to develop meaningful care plans and prioritize problem areas.

At this point, the hypothesis was confirmed and the task identified. The nursing admission assessment form needed to be redesigned.

Plan

After identifying the problem, I developed a vision for a new nursing assessment form. It needed to be user friendly for the nursing staff, yet functional. From this vision, I developed preliminary goals for the new nursing admission form:

- Reader-friendly horizontal flow
- Logical flow so that similar items are grouped together
- Documentation requirements must be reduced
- Flow must lead to prompts to remind the nurse of the important items to address
- Accreditation requirements must be interwoven in natural flow within the context of the assessment and become more meaningful components to the assessment
- Typesetting must be professional
- Cheerful colors must be incorporated to provide more pleasure for the users
- An overall summary section must be easy for team members to review

Because of the short time frame and because the responsibility to succeed with this aspect of the JCAHO survey was on my shoulders, I chose not to delegate the project, but to assume its leadership.

I began by researching published admission assessment forms, looking for user-friendly formats, standard assessment processes, and summary sections. A basic format that would provide the framework for the new assessment form was the nurse admission form used at Ashland Community Hospital in Ashland, OR.[1] This form contained basic elements identified in the first three original goals, such as horizontal layout, logical flow, and reduced documentation requirements. This format also would serve as a great springboard for incorporation of the remaining goals for the new nursing assessment, such as prompts, interwoven accreditation requirements, cheerful colors, and a summary section. I began by drafting a sample page of the new assessment form. This started the process of active feedback and an information exchange between the nurse managers and myself. As draft pages were developed, the team was continually consulted. This process was critically important because the nurse managers were advocates for the entire nursing staff, and input of the staff and managers was essential before I proceeded to the next sections.

As the nursing assessment form took shape, nursing topics were grouped together in sections that flowed logically together. I decided to use a basic format that was developed with negative findings so that the nurse only needed to indicate negative exceptions to a healthy assessment. I believed that this would minimize charting and clarify problematic areas in the patient's assessment. If a section was normal, a quick check box indicating "no problems noted" was provided. Assessment fields and criteria were changed to better address the type of patients seen at our hospital.

To incorporate the goal of prompts, I added a prompt box to each body system section. It was developed for the nurse to mark if there were negative findings and if the findings should be considered for the care plan. In addition, for increased connection to the care plan, each prompt box included the corresponding problem number from the care plan.

To further refine the form, I grouped together the need for financial assistance, need for case management referral, spiritual considerations, suspected abuse and neglect, and assistance at home, as well as other regulatory issues. I placed prompt boxes by these sections because it was the team's belief that referrals to case management, the business office, and social services were also important in care planning. Such referrals or at least the documentation of the referral, had often times been missing on our old assessment form. Because referrals are an important part of providing comprehensive patient care, we wanted to ensure that other disciplines were appropriately notified based on the individual patient findings. Interestingly, we generated so many referrals to wound management, we had to rethink our referral criteria to ensure that only patients requiring the expertise of a wound specialist were referred. Many of the skin and wound issues were a component of standard nursing care and could be addressed through the nursing plan of care.

A big challenge in the development of the form was the need to incorporate regulatory requirements into the sections to which they were related, in order to improve their meaningfulness. For instance, was it better to include the functional trigger assessment layout provided by the physical therapy department with the musculoskeletal system or with the neurological system? Should the fall-risk assessment follow or precede the musculoskeletal section? Would the nutritional trigger assessment layout provided by the dietitians be best with the gastrointestinal system assessment or would it be best in a separate section? And, where would the spiritual considerations be most meaningful in the context of the assessment? And, should some items, such as the learning assessment, be removed from the assessment and relocated to another more pertinent form?

The team helped answer each of these questions on a preliminary basis. The final answers would come later, after staff began reviewing and using the form, but first drafts of the form had to be prepared for them to review.

Another significant principle in redesigning the form was that nurses deserve to work with forms that are easy to read and feature cheerful colors. This conviction guided my overall development of the form. I developed sections with ease of the reader in mind, and the team chose cheerful colors to divide sections and to accentuate and differentiate prompt boxes for referrals, care planning, and miscellaneous items. For the inpatient admission assessment, the team chose a yellow highlight to divide sections. The prompt boxes for care planning were also highlighted in yellow. Prompt boxes for referrals were highlighted in green, and miscellaneous prompt boxes were highlighted in lavender.

The final section of the nursing admission assessment was developed to serve as the final summary for the assessment. The purpose of this section was to provide a summary of the assessment in a way that any viewer could find the essential findings with ease. Each summary-box topic was listed in the final summary section in its corresponding color. The intent of this section was for the nurse to scan back through the entire admission assessment, review each sectional prompt box, and record a final assessment summary. It was also designed so that the top three care plan topics would be identified for initial care planning. This would help the nurses prioritize the patient's problems and choose those most meaningful for initial care. It was our intent to have the nurses focus on problems that could reasonably be addressed during their hospital stay. We discouraged inclusion of multiple potential problems as our shortened length of stay required us to concentrate on the actual issues that led to the patient's hospitalization.

After an initial draft was developed and reviewed by the nurse managers, it was time for more nursing staff involvement. The form was presented to the facility's Nursing Leadership Group (NLG), a group made up of nursing staff leaders who meet monthly to address nursing-related issues. The group reviewed the form and provided feedback. They endorsed the form and two members volunteered to conduct pilots on their nursing units. During the pilot period, the volunteers recorded desired modifications to a master copy of the form. We were committed to responding to revisions recommended by the nurses and therefore we chose to obtain their input and change the form until the tool could be refined to the nurse's satisfaction. At the conclusion of the pilot, the NLG met again and formalized their recommendations. The nurse managers and I were pleased to learn that the desired modifications were minor.

Implementation

The NLG participated in the rollout of the new nursing assessment form in June 2005, just a month and a half after our consultant's visit. One of the NLG members volunteered to lead training sessions for all nursing staff. I attended the meetings to support the NLG leader conducting the training and also to be present to answer questions that might have to do with the background theory behind the form. The majority of the nursing staff attended the sessions and provided additional feedback and questions.

Once again, I integrated the suggested modifications into the form and considered and addressed questions that arose about charting by exception and prioritization of care-plan issues. One concern that came up while speaking with the nurses was the change to charting by exception. Several nurses were concerned about their liability with only charting the negatives. They felt much safer documenting a full assessment even if the findings were normal. Based on their concerns, I consulted our attorney. We discussed the form and the theory behind charting by exception, and he concluded that he was comfortable with this style of charting. To help the nurses feel even more comfortable, I wrote a policy that addressed this style of charting on the assessment so they would have a policy to back them up in the event their charting was reviewed.

Once the training sessions were completed and staff issues addressed, the form was initiated on all nursing units. A copy of the final form can be found at the end of this chapter.

As for the questions that arose about how to incorporate regulatory requirements into the sections to which they were related to help increase their meaningfulness, the staff provided feedback about where to best place these sections. The functional trigger assessment was found to be most meaningful when placed after the neurological and musculoskeletal sections because information learned in both of these assessments helped assess functional status. The fall-risk assessment that was once tacked on at the end of our admission assessment was incorporated into the assessment just following the functional assessment because information gained in the functional assessment was relevant to the fall assessment. We felt that coordinating this type of information gathering creates a natural flow for the nurse.

The nutritional trigger assessment could be placed in several locations, but we chose to place it just following the GI section because we felt this location better connected the GI assessment to the history. When assessing spiritual considerations, we felt it was best to add it to the first page and include it in our psychosocial/economic/discharge section where information about home, finances, and other social-service related issues were assessed. And finally, we evaluated miscellaneous items on our assessment to see if there was a better place to incorporate the information. For instance, the advance directive questions were revised and reassigned to the admitting office because we felt this was a better venue for collecting the information. Our learning assessment was relocated to our teaching sheet so that each nurse could refer to the assessment information when preparing to teach the patient rather than having to refer back to the admission assessment.

Evaluation

The staff provided favorable feedback about the new assessment process, stating that they liked it and that it saved them time, some reporting that it saved them 20 minutes per assessment. One of the nurse auditors at our facility has said that the form helps her when she's looking for compliance with regulatory issues. She says the items are easier to find and she too enjoys the clear print and pleasant colors. And agency staff members provided input that the form was so easy to use that little, if any, orientation was necessary to complete the nursing assessment. The new form was so successful that the pediatric nurses in our facility requested and received a new pediatric admission assessment in a similar format.

Melody Thames, an RN charge nurse for the telemetry unit, best sums up the benefits of the new form from the perspective of a staff nurse: "As any other nurse, my time is crunched. I found that this admit form dropped 15 to 20 minutes off any admit, and the triggers brought up questions not normally remembered, saving my brain power for other problems."

Jean Wallace, RN, charge nurse for the medical unit, agrees. "The work of admitting patients has been simplified greatly with this assessment tool," she says. "Each problem that is addressed with the patient is simplified by either choosing that problem and checking the questions that are listed or by simply checking the 'no problem' square. Each problem is color coded with the nursing diagnosis list which makes the process of choosing nursing diagnoses for each patient's individual needs simpler."

The true test of whether our new form met the original goal of improving care planning came when our consultant returned for her follow-up visit. She said she found it to be an excellent tool, and she observed chart reviews that indicated a significant improvement in completed assessment and care planning. The nursing staff were very positive and proud of their accomplishments and could easily speak to the patient's care needs identified during the assessment process.

The next test was our facility's JCAHO survey in July 2005, and again our form passed with flying colors. The surveyors were very impressed with our admission assessment form, and the physician surveyor liked it so much he asked for a copy to take with him when he left. And as a result, we concluded that our efforts had greatly improved the meaningfulness, accuracy, and updating of care plans.

Conclusion

The development of this assessment form was a strenuous process—especially with the short turn-around time we had before our JCAHO survey in July. However, it was extremely rewarding to collaborate with the staff nurses and create a tool that not only helps them complete their work more efficiently, but also is more pleasant to look at and use each and every day. Truly, the heart of this process was working together with the staff, garnering their input, ideas, and criticism, and then integrating this feedback into a form everyone was comfortable using.

1   Anne Griffin Perry and Patricia A. Potter, *Clinical Nursing Skills & Technique*, 5th ed.   (St. Louis, Missouri: Mosby, 2003), 42.

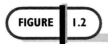 **FIGURE** **1.2**

Current patient admission assessment record

Part I: Admission Routine		
Date: **Time:**	**T:** **P:** **R:** **O₂ Sat:**	
Mode: ☐ amb ☐ gurney ☐ w/c ☐ other	**B/P:** Rt Lt:	
Via: ☐ admitting ☐ ER ☐ OR ☐ other	**Height:** **Weight:** ☐Stand ☐Bed ☐Stated	

Admitting MD: **Family MD:**

Admitting Diagnosis:

Chief Complaint: (per patient)

Allergies: ☐ NKDA	**Latex:** ☐ balloons ☐ bananas ☐ gloves ☐ pineapple	**LATEX** 4 or > - order latex free cart ☐
Type of Reaction:	☐ mult OR ☐ avocados	
Valuables List: (describe jewelry, clothing, etc.)		**VALUABLE** envelope to Safe ☐
☐ Glasses ☐ Contact lenses ☐ Dentures ☐ Partial/bridge ☐ Hearing aid ☐ Refused safe		

Nurse Signature (if other than nurse completing remainder of assessment):

Part II: Patient History		

Patient History: (major illnesses/operations/major injuries)

☐ Hypertension	☐ COPD	☐ Diabetes	☐ Cancer	☐ Anesthesia issues
☐ Heart Disease	☐ Asthma	☐ Hepatitis	☐ Seizures	☐ None
☐ Stroke	☐ TB	☐ Ulcer	☐ Mental Disorder	
☐ Cardiac other	☐ Respiratory other	☐ Kidney Disease	☐ General other	

To OR & anesthesia issue HX; call MD ☐

Specify others not listed above and Surgeries:

SMOKING & yes to MI, Pneu, CHF; give Ed. ☐

Alcohol/Drug Use: ☐ Yes ☐ No	Type:	Daily Amt:	☐ Quit
Tobacco Use: ☐ Yes ☐ No	Type:	Daily Amt:	☐ Quit
Admitting Diagnosis: AMI, Pneumonia, CHF:	☐ Yes ☐ No		

FLU/PNEU If no, do Screen form ☐

Vaccinations:

Flu Shot within past 12 months	☐ Yes	☐ No	☐ Refused
Pneumonia Shot in past 5 years	☐ Yes	☐ No	☐ Refused

CM Flu/Pneu Referral ☐

Family History:

☐ Heart Disease	☐ Hypertension	☐ Stroke	☐ Asthma	☐ TB	☐ Diabetes	☐ Kidney	☐ Anesthesia
☐ Cancer	☐ Seizures	☐ Blood Disorder	☐ Mental Disorder	☐ None	☐ Other:		

Psychosocial/Economic/Discharge:

Marital Status: ☐ Married ☐ Single ☐ Widowed	**FINANCE** Referral ☐
Family: ☐ Lives With ☐ Lives Alone	
Lives In: ☐ Home ☐ Nursing Home ☐ Other	
Occupation: ☐ Full Time ☐ Part Time ☐ Retired ☐ Other	**SS or CM** Referral ☐
Requests Visit from Business Office Rep or HELP Program ☐ Yes ☐ No	
Activity Level: ☐ Ambulatory ☐ Cane ☐ Walker ☐ Wheelchair ☐ Bedrest	
Suspected Abuse/Neglect: ☐ Yes ☐ No	
Emotional Status: ☐ Cooperative ☐ Anxious ☐ Depressed ☐ End of Life	**ANXIETY** ☐ poc#1
Concerns with Hospitalization: ☐ Child Care ☐ Home Life ☐ Religious/Cultural Practices	**GRIEF** ☐ poc #2 **KNOW DEF** ☐ poc #3
Emergency Contact: POA: ☐ yes ☐ no Relation: Phone:	**SPIRITUAL** ☐ poc #4
Nearest Relative: Relation: Phone:	
Info. Obtained from: ☐ Patient ☐ Family ☐ Other	

Page 1 of 4   Patient Label

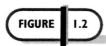

FIGURE 1.2

Current patient admission assessment record (cont.)

Part III: Physical Assessment (Place a check in areas of abnormality. If unable to assess, indicate reason.)

Assess eyes, ears, nose, for abnormality ☐ **No Problem Noted**

EENT					
☐ impaired vision	☐ glaucoma	☐ hard of hearing	☐ gums	☐ redness	☐ drainage
☐ blind		☐ deaf	☐ teeth	☐ burning	☐ lesion

Notes:

EENT: POC ☐

Assess chest configuration, resp. rate, depth, pattern, breath sounds ☐ **No Problem Noted**

RESPIRATORY					
☐ asymmetric	☐ tachypnea	☐ crackles	Right: ☐ up ☐ low Left: ☐ up ☐ low	☐ cough
☐ barrel chest	☐ bradypnea	☐ diminished	Right: ☐ up ☐ low Left: ☐ up ☐ low	☐ sputum-color
☐ dyspnea	☐ shallow	☐ wheezes	Right: ☐ up ☐ low Left: ☐ up ☐ low	O₂ @ ___ liters/min

Notes:

RESP: poc#6 ☐

Assess heart rate, pulse, blood pressure, circulation, fluid retention ☐ **No Problem Noted**

CARDIO VASCULAR				
☐ tachycardia	☐ irregular	☐ tingling	☐ edema	☐ diminished pulses:
☐ bradycardia	☐ murmur	☐ numbness	☐ fatigue	☐ absent pulses:

Notes:

CardioV: poc#7 ☐

Assess abdomen, bowel sounds, bowel habits ☐ **No Problem Noted**

GASTRO INTESTINAL					
☐ distention	☐ hypo BS	☐ anorexia	☐ dysphagic	☐ diarrhea	☐ incontinent
☐ rigidity	☐ hyper BS	☐ N or V	☐ constipation	☐ last BM :	☐ ostomy
☐ special diet		☐ diet intolerances		☐ diabetes	

Notes:

GI: ☐ poc #8 or #9 **Endocrine** poc #10 **Nutrition** poc #11 ☐

Nutritional Trigger Assessment: ☐ **No Problem Noted**

NUTRITION		
☐ weight change > 10lb within the last month	☐ decubitus - stage II or greater
☐ changes in appetite/intake > 3 days	☐ TPN/tube feeding/PEG tube
☐ N/V/diarrhea > 3 days	☐ DX: malnutrition, FTT, or Gest DM

Dietary Trigger ☐ Referral:

Assess urine frequency, control (Gyn - assess bleeding, discharge, pregnancy) ☐ **No Problem Noted**

GU and GYN					
☐ dysuria	☐ hesitancy	☐ nocturia	☐ foley	☐ menopausal	☐ discharge
☐ frequency	☐ incontinent	☐ hematuria	☐ urostomy	☐ LMP	☐ pregnancy

Notes:

GU & GYN: poc#12 ☐

Page 2 of 4 | Patient Label

Nursing Assessment, Plan of Care, and Patient Education: The Foundation of Patient Care

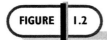 **FIGURE** **1.2**

Current patient admission assessment record (cont.)

Part III: Physical Assessment (Place a check in areas of abnormality. If unable to assess, indicate reason.)

Assess orientation, LOC, speech, strength, grip, ☐ **No Problem Noted**

☐ confused	☐ sedated	☐ pupil/Lt. non react	☐ vertigo	☐ tremors	☐ unsteady
☐ comatose	☐ lethargic	☐ aphasic	☐ headaches	☐ numbness	☐ paralyzed
☐ semi-comatose	☐ pupil/Rt. non react	☐ slurred speech	☐ seizures	☐ tingling	☐ grips - weak

NEURO

Notes:

NEURO: POC ☐

Assess mobility, joint function, skin color, turgor, integrity ☐ **No Problem Noted**

☐ appliance	☐ swelling	☐ diaphoretic	☐ moist
☐ prosthesis	☐ skin color	☐ hot	☐ flushed
☐ deformity/atrophy	☐ poor turgor	☐ cool	☐ drainage

MS & SKIN

Notes:

SKIN ISSUES: Wd Care Referral ☐

MS: POC ☐

Norton Scale (Skin Risk Assessment)

Reprinted with permission: Doreen Norton, Rhoda McLaren, and A.N. Exton-Smith, An Investigation of Geriatric Nursing Problems in Hospitals. National Corporation for the Care of Old People (now Centre for Policy on Ageing). London. 1962.

Physical Condition	1. Very bad	2. Poor	3. Fair	4. Good	
Mental Condition	1. Stupor	2. Confused	3. Apathetic	4. Alert	
Activity	1. Bed	2. Chair Bound	3. Walk Help	4. Ambulant	
Mobility	1. Immobile	2. Very Limited	3. Slightly Limited	4. Full	
Incontinence	1. Doubly	2. Usually/Urine	3. Occasional	4. Not	
Notes:		If 14 or less, evaluate appropriateness for Plan of Care.		**Total Score**	

NORTON SCALE

SKIN: poc#15 ☐

Functional Trigger Assessment:

		Usual ADL	**Admit ADL**	**Total Score = Usual-Admit**
Code:	**OT** feeds self/dressing/ADLs			
4 = 100% of care	**PT** gait/transfers			
3 = 75% of care	**ST** swallow/expression/comprehension			
2 = 50% of care			**ADL:** poc# 16 ☐	**FUNCTION:** Referral to Phys. Med. if change ☐
1 = 25% of care				
0 = N/A - (acute time limited condition)				

FUNCTION

Fall Risk (Risk Assessment)

☐ **Level I**	☐ **Level II** - *Has two or more of the following risk factors*
any patient	☐ age >65
	☐ history of falls (immed or within past 3 mo.)
	☐ taking fall related medications (hypnotics, analgesics, psychotropics, antihypertensive, diuretic, laxative)
	☐ mod to severe physical impairment (includes mobility or visual/hearing deficits)
	☐ occasional or frequent cognitive impairment

FALL RISK

FALL RISK II: poc#17 ☐

Page 3 of 4

Patient label

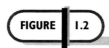

FIGURE 1.2 **Current patient admission assessment record (cont.)**

Brownwood Regional Medical Center	Patient Admission Assessment Record

Part III: Physical Assessment (Place a check in areas of abnormality. If unable to assess, indicate reason.)

Pain Assessment

PAIN					
pain score =	☐ numbers (A)	☐ faces (B)	☐ FLACC (C)		Pain goal:
location:					☐ Unable to give
onset:					
variations:					
quality:	☐ ache	☐ dull	☐ sharp	☐ stabbing	☐ throbbing
	☐ cramping	☐ burning	☐ shooting	☐ pressure	☐ other:
aggravates:	☐ light	☐ dark	☐ movement	☐ lying down	☐ other
relieves:	☐ eating	☐ quiet	☐ cold	☐ heat	☐ other
medications:					
effects of pain:	☐ N/V	☐ sleep	☐ appetite	☐ activity	**PAIN:** poc#18
	☐ relationships	☐ emotions	☐ other		☐

Home Medications (list medication, dose and frequency, and last dose taken)

MEDICATIONS	Medication:	Dose/Freq.:	Last Dose:	Medication:	Dose/Freq.:	Last Dose:
	☐ Refer to printed NH med list with last dose identified			☐ Refer to cont. med sheet w/ last dose identified		

Disposition of Medications:	☐ *did not bring*	☐ *to pharmacy*	☐ *family to take home*
Medication Sheet faxed to pharmacy:	☐ *yes*		

Admission Summary/Plan:

SUMMARY	General:	Referrals:	Plan of Care: Choose top 3 priorities for Plan of Care			
	☐ Latex Cart	☐ CM/SS Ref.	☐ Anxiety #1	☐ Cardio V. #7	☐ GU/Gyn #12	☐ Infection #19
	☐ Valuables	☐ Finance Ref.	☐ Grief #2	☐ GI #8 (alterations)	☐ Skin #15	☐ Other #20
	☐ Smoking Ed.	☐ Nutrition Ref.	☐ Know Def. #3	☐ GI #9 (fluid/volume)	☐ ADL #16	
	☐ Flu/Pneu Scre	☐ Wound Ref.	☐ Spiritual #4	☐ Endocrine #10	☐ Fall/injury #17	
		☐ Phys M Ref.	☐ Resp. #6	☐ Nutrition #11	☐ Pain #18	

Date:	Time:	RN Signature:
Page 4 of 4		Patient label

    Nursing Assessment, Plan of Care, and Patient Education: The Foundation of Patient Care

Case Study #1 One hospital's journey to developing a multidisciplinary assessment form

In the United States, it's estimated that, on average, a patient comes in contact with as many as 50 caregivers during the first 24 hours of admission.[1] Before a task force at the Presbyterian Medical Center in Phialdephia, PA developed a multidisciplinary assessment form, patients in the oncology unit complained that during their return visits several caregivers asked about their alleged history. They began to wonder if anyone in the hospital bothered to read the patient charts or talk to one another. Administrators and team members decided to streamline the admission care process so that one person could ask questions from a form that all disciplines could use as a reference. A single form would not only reduce the workload, but also prevent caregivers from asking patients the same questions during the first 24 to 48 hours of their hospital stay.

Getting started

Hospital leaders fully supported the concept of developing an integrated patient assessment form in 1992 when Presbyterian Medical Center received a deficiency on the medical record documentation portion of its Joint Commission on Accreditation of Healthcare Organizations (JCAHO) survey. Surveyors suggested that the hospital consolidate the questions on existing forms used to document initial patient information. They also recommended that caregivers from different disciplines start using the data physicians and nurses collect at admission.

In 1994, team members from patient care services (nursing, physical therapy, nutrition, social work, respiratory care, and pharmacy) created an integrated patient admission assessment tool based on the hospital's nursing assessment form. This form gathered information germane to all patient service departments. However, this document was never tested on inpatient units because the medical staff revamped its standardized history and physical form (H&P) at the same time the team developed the new assessment form.

The original H&P asked physicians to fill in a blank form based on guidelines established by the medical staff. However, physicians usually completed the form based on their own individual needs. Since Presbyterian is a teaching facility, the medical staff argued that the standardized H&P was more appropriate than the integrated assessment tool because it helped train interns and residents on what types of information they need to collect upon a patient's admission.

This information, such as physical assessments, immunization, code status, nutrition, and social history is especially important because interns and residents will have to ask these questions in private practice. Although it's a legitimate argument, in reality, residents, interns, and house staff don't always ask the questions. Instead, they decide what questions to ask based on the patient's immediate care needs and their own time limitations.

Even though the standardized H&P meant the integrated assessment tool was set aside, the form actually helped pave the way for physicians to understand the benefit of a multidisciplinary assessment form. The H&P was comprehensive, but it still duplicated many of the questions that nurses asked during the assessment.

Patient care team members eventually garnered support for the multidisciplinary assessment projects when consultants were hired by the hospital to help the staff prepare for the 1995 JCAHO survey. The consultants saw a draft of the form and liked the concept. Medical staff leaders began to understand the benefits of the form after the hospital reviewed hundreds of records as part of its survey preparation. Leaders noticed that physicians wrote simple paragraphs in the H&P instead of a comprehensive review. Many physicians also wrote "refer to nursing assessment form" under certain sections of the H&P instead of entering the data.

Renewed interest in the form occurred during the actual survey when patient care team members showed surveyors a prototype of the integrated patient assessment form. Surveyors were impressed. The chief of the residency program and the president of the medical staff later reconsidered the idea for a multidisciplinary assessment form and agreed to serve on the task force to help develop it.

Securing upper management support

The first order of business when undertaking any project is securing upper management support. Fortunately, the culture at Presbyterian encourages and supports cooperation among departments; the medical administration works closely with the nursing administration. As a result, the core team members found support early in the process. Upper management believed in the concept that several disciplines working together provides the best possible care for patients. They were willing to support the development of the form as a way to improve patient satisfaction and documentation.

However, it's important to note that the project easily could stall if one of its supporters leaves the hospital for another position. This actually occurred at Presbyterian when the project chair left midway through the process. The task force fortunately had someone equally respected by the medical staff to take over as project chair. Before embarking on a project of this magnitude, make sure both upper management and key medical staff support it. Without their blessing, this project will not be successful.

Setting up the task force

Once Presbyterian's upper management supported the project, the core team members selected representatives from other disciplines to join the task force to review the draft form. The core team included the director of nursing for medical/surgical and ambulatory care, the director of nursing for perioperative and critical care, the president of the medical staff, and the quality improvement coordinator for patient care services.

Other task force members included physicians, nurses, and representatives from social work, physical therapy, nutrition, medical records, and respiratory care. In addition to the president of the medical staff, the physicians who served on the team included the head of the residency program, a pulmonologist, and the head of quality management for the medical staff.

Developing the first drafts of the form

The core team members created the first draft of the form before showing it to the entire task force. It didn't take long to come up with the original draft. Since the hospital already had excellent nursing assessment and physician H&P forms, the team merged the best of both forms to create a new document. Designing the form was simply a matter of cutting out the best sections from both documents and pasting them together. All the questions chosen to remain on the new form addressed JCAHO standard requirements.

The entire task force met to review the draft document. It only took one or two meetings over the course of three months for the task force to decide the format and content of the tool. The process flowed smoothly. Discussions centered on the order of the questions and whether to include certain questions. For instance, the team considered eliminating questions related to immunizations since physicians frequently didn't fill out this section on the H&P. The physicians on the task force wanted to include the questions because in some cases it's important to know the patient's immunization history. The immunization questions remained, but the section included a "not applicable" checkbox. If physicians check the "not applicable" box, it indicates they at least considered the immunization history instead of just leaving the section blank. It also demonstrates to JCAHO surveyors that physicians are evaluating the patient's immunization history if the information is pertinent.

After this review process, task force members took the form back to their departments for a staff review. The department of nutrition fine-tuned the nutritional questions addressed under the nursing assessment section. Physical therapists reviewed functional status questions. Social service and psychiatry added their thoughts on questions about coping and family involvement. Respiratory therapists made sure the form included questions about the patient's history of respiratory or pulmonary problems. Physicians made suggestions on the sections that covered the review of systems and physical exam. This staff review ensured the new form addressed the assessment needs of all caregivers.

Physicians have free space to record their impressions during the initial assessment. However, the nursing assessment section consists of check-off boxes and grids. The nursing section is unique because it includes a question that asks if the nurse has identified a patient's learning needs. A follow-up question asks whether the patient wants consultative services or additional information.
After completing the staff review, the task force needed only to decide who completes each section of the form and the layout of the form needed to be finalized. The group ultimately decided that the front page should contain information that all disciplines need to know immediately—chief compliaint, primary physician, code status, history of present illnesses, medications, and allergies. The team designed the rest of the form in order of importance as a way to encourage caregivers to complete all the sections without jumping pages. Physicians fill out sections shaded gray. Nursing sections are white.

During the final discussions about the form, the team agreed to eliminate questions or change the layout if the caregivers who used the form during the proposed pilot study didn't like the format or noticed the form included similar questions in more than one section.

By the time the task force agreed on the final version, the business form company contracted by the hospital had created eight drafts for the team to review.

Selling the idea to staff

Developing the form is one important step, getting physicians to believe in the project is another. Despite upper management's support, it took nearly a year to get enough physicians on board to run a pilot study.

Even though the majority of the medical staff was convinced that the integrated form was the way to go after the survey, doubters still remained. Some physicians were uncomfortable with the form. A few wanted to make sure they could still ask the same open-ended questions they asked on the standardized H&P form. Others expressed concern that a nurse may have the assessment form when other personnel need to use it. Several physicians argued that the new form would make it easier for JCAHO surveyors to spot deficiencies. For instance, they believed surveyors would notice immediately if they left questions about a patient's visual history blank. They thought the old narrative form made it more difficult to locate such missing information.

Physicians on the task force had to persuade their peers that the form was beneficial. They tried to sell the idea of the form to the rest of the medical staff. They discussed it at department meetings, in the hallways, and at noontime conferences for the house staff. Because the medical staff admired and respected the physician leaders on the task force, they eventually agreed to test the form in a pilot study.

Preparing for the pilot study

To determine if caregivers could work with the multidisciplinary assessment form, the task force prepared to test the form in three different patient care areas. However, the medical executive committee wanted to keep the pilot small and controlled, so members agreed to conduct the pilot on two patient care units. The goal was to complete 50 forms in three months.

The pilot program

Presbyterian Medical Center of the University of Pennsylvania Health System is a 355-bed community tertiary care facility. The three-month pilot program began in September 1996. The task force's goal was to use the forms on a total of 50 patients admitted to either the same-day surgery unit or the acute care of elders unit during the pilot program. The task force and medical executive committee selected these units to ensure a small, controlled study using the same house staff and nurse practitioners.

The team used the pilot as a way to identify which sections of the form worked well and which sections needed improvement. If, at the conclusion of the trial, physicians and nurses liked the form, the hospital intended to introduce the document to various units until the tool was used hospital-wide. Administrators at the University of Pennsylvania Medical Center, another hospital in the University of Pennsylvania Health System, were also interested in the multidisciplinary assessment form, but they wanted to see first how the form worked hospital-wide at Presbyterian before implementing it system-wide.

Education

The Department of Nursing taught 34 staff members (two nurse practitioners, 20 nurses, and 12 house staff) how to use the form before the team implemented the pilot program. The training sessions varied in time and instruction. Nurses on each shift of the acute care of elders unit only required an hour of instruction because the multidisciplinary form is similar to the nursing patient admission assessment form. The instruction included an explanation of the changes and which section the nurses needed to complete. Trainers also discussed potential problems, such as the conflict that could arise if a physician needed the chart while a nurse was using it.

House staff and nurse practitioners received more detailed instruction. Nurse practitioners must complete all eight pages of the form, while physicians are only required to complete its shaded areas. Instructors explained the philosophy behind the form, the reasons the house staff and nurse practitioners were selected for the pilot program, and the importance of completing the entire form. Instructors also described the form's benefits to both caregivers and patients. House staff received training each month during the pilot study because of rotation schedules.

Other departments—such as respiratory, physical therapy, and nutrition—received a brief overview because they only used the form for reference and the new multidisciplinary assessment form was similar to the previous nursing assessment tool.

The results

The staff completed 50 pilot forms and the team reviewed 30 of the charts. Staff in the acute care of elders unit completed nine admission assessment charts. The same-day surgery unit completed the remaining 21 charts.

The task force was pleased with the initial results. In several instances, doctors, nurses, and nurse practitioners achieved 100% compliance when filling out the form. Please refer to Figure A.1 for a summary of the pilot findings.

For a comparison of the pilot program findings to the number of charts completed using the former nursing assessment tool and standardized H&P, see Figure A.2

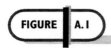

Results of the pilot program

The following data are based on completion of 30 patient charts. The statistics include the number of charts completed in both the same-day surgery unit and the acute elderly care unit, and the percentage of compliance for each section of the form.

Nursing sections	TOTAL	PERCENTAGE
Medications	20	97
Allergies	30	100
Substance abuse	29	97
Nutritional/metabolic	29	97
Elimination	29	97
Activity/exercise	29	97
Sleep/rest	29	97
Sexuality/reproductive	22	73
Cognitive/perceptual	29	97
Coping/stress	29	97
Value/belief	29	97
Role/relationship	25	83
Skin assessment	25	83
Summation questions	28	93
Notations made when section is not applicable or unable to be attained	13	43
Nurses documented the date and time they started working on the form	30	100
Signature, date, and time nurses completed the section	26	87
Physician/Nurse practitioner sections		
Primary care MD	26	90
Chief complaint	27	93
Hx present illness	29	100
Past medical Hx	29	100
Family Hx	29	100
Review of systems	26	90
Immunizations	26	90
Physical exam	29	100
Initial diagnostics	22	76
Summary	29	100
Admitting Dx	29	100
Tx plan	29	100
Date, time, beeper, and printed name of physician/NP	25	83
Physician/Nurse practitioner signature	30	100

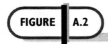

FIGURE A.2

Comparison data

The following data reflect how well the nursing and physician staffs complied with documentation using the former nursing assessment form and the standardized H&P. It is based on the completion of 30 patient assessment forms. The percentages reflect compliance with each section of the form. See **Figure A.1** to compare the results.

Nursing sections	TOTAL	PERCENTAGE
Medications	28	93
Allergies	29	97
Substance abuse	30	100
Nutritional/metabolic	29	97
Elimination	30	100
Activity/exercise	30	100
Sleep/rest	30	100
Sexuality/reproductive	29	97
Cognitive/perceptual	30	100
Coping/stress	29	97
Value/belief	29	97
Role/relationship	29	97
Skin assessment	28	93
Summation questions	28	93
Notations made when section is not applicable or unable to be attained	22	73
Nurses documented the date and time they started working on the form	28	93
Signature, date, and time nurses completed the section	25	83
Physician/Nurse practitioner sections		
Primary care MD	12	40
Chief complaint	28	93
Hx present illness	29	97
Past medical Hx	28	93
Family Hx	22	73
Review of systems	24	80
Immunizations	13	43
Physical exam	29	97
Initial diagnostics	27	90
Summary	29	97
Admitting Dx	24	80
Tx plan	24	80
Date, time, beeper, and printed name of physician/NP	23	77
Physician/Nurse practitioner signature	26	97

The pilot program also identified poor compliance with the "not applicable" or "unable to obtain" checkboxes. Instead of checking off the box, staff members left the section blank. Task force members intend to ask staff for suggestions to help improve compliance. Before the hospital expanded the pilot, the task force incorporated the suggestions made by staff members into a new version of the form.

Recommendations

Throughout the pilot program, the team asked the participants for both verbal and written comments. In general, they liked the form, and found it self-explanatory and easy to use. However, nurse practitioners—the only ones who fill out the entire eight-page document—thought the form was too long. Nurse practitioners also noticed that both the nursing and physician sections included questions about female patients' menstrual history, last Pap smear, and mammogram. The task force reviewed these two sections and rearranged the questions.

Before the pilot began, physicians expected to run into hand-off problems with nurses over the patient charts. Although it's possible a nurse and physician could want to gather the data at the same time, physicians on the acute care of elders unit reported it wasn't a problem. Nurses usually completed the assessment before the physician arrived on the floor. One physician didn't want to rely on the nurse's assessment and completed the entire section, but this was the exception. Most physicians referred to the nursing assessment section for information.

Nurses also reported few problems. Some had a difficult time adjusting to the fact they no longer have the option to "defer" sections if a patient is unresponsive or the question isn't applicable. Unlike the previous nursing assessment tool, the new form requires them to document why the patient is unable to respond to the questions or why it's not applicable.

Many participants didn't like the design of the assessment form. They complained the pull-out or spreadsheet design made it difficult to complete when writing on a clipboard. As a result, physicians had trouble referring to their notes from previous pages, and nurses found it easy to miss entire sections because of the pull-out format. Task force members changed the design of the form before it was piloted in other areas.

Summary

When the form is eventually used throughout the hospital, training will be more intense. The nursing department will sponsor mandatory noontime conferences, create posters, and visit each unit to explain the changes.

1. Lathrop, J.P. *Restructuring Health Care: The Patient Focused Paradigm*, San Francisco, Jossey-Bass, 1993.

Source: Seltzer, B.L., Brodrick, T.M., Magner, J.J., How to *Develop and Implement a Multidisciplinary Assessment Form*, Marblehead, MA, Opus Communications, 1997.

Case Study #2: Experimental admission and discharge teams improve throughput and staff satisfaction

Emergency Department overcrowding, complex cases, prolonged length of story, nurses paralyzed by paperwork, hospital bottlenecks . . . does this describe your facility? Two experimental pilot programs prove that implementing an admission and discharge team may help ease some of these common, yet debilitating problems.

San Jacinto Methodist Hospital (SJMH) in Baytown, TX launched a new pilot program called DART. The program is designed to support SJMH's medical and surgical areas with aspects of the nursing process that are time consuming, particularly the admission and discharge of patients.

When the decision is made to admit a patient from the ED, DART nurses go to the patient while he or she is still in the ED to begin the initial assessment. They may also begin the admission process when a patient is transferred from the ED to his or her room or is a direct admission.

"The overall goal is to improve patient care [and] productivity and to heighten patient, nurse, and physician satisfaction," says **Elizabeth Heil, RN, MS,** manager of nursing resources and informatics at SJMH.

"The program started on a unit where patient satisfaction scores were way down, but two months after implementing DART, our Press Ganey scores were significantly better," she says.

During admission, a DART nurse receives a page of information from the admitting office or a report from the ED, greets the patient, and completes the initial admission assessment process. The DART nurse also begins the discharge planning form at the time of admission, as appropriate, and coordinates initial consults with the ostomy nurse, diabetic director, or any other specialists who may be needed, says Heil.

The DART nurse also provides education to the patient and family to ensure understanding of the discharge instructions and medications. DART nurses spend a minimum of 30 minutes on a discharge with a patient, printing medication lists and instructions and allowing time for questions. "Before, a floor nurse would say, 'I can do a discharge in five to 10 minutes,' " says Heil. "Well, that's exactly what the problem was."

    Nursing Assessment, Plan of Care, and Patient Education: The Foundation of Patient Care

As part of the comprehensive discharge planning process, DART nurses also place follow-up calls to patients 24 hours after discharge to determine

- how the patient is doing at home
- if the patient is experiencing any problems
- how the patient felt about the care provided
- what improvements could be made

During the phone call, a DART nurse reinforces discharge teaching and asks patients whether there are any staff members that deserve recognition. If a patient identifies an issue or wants to recognize a caregiver, it is the DART nurse's responsibility to ensure that follow-up occurs.

"Administration particularly likes this aspect of the program because it connects the patient to the hospital community," says Heil. Nurses, nurse technicians, case managers, and doctors have all been recognized by patients through this process. When staff are recognized three times, they receive a star on their certificates. "No money is involved, but you would be surprised how much this incentive boosts morale," she says. "It is a great motivator."

Currently, two DART nurses work between 7 a.m. and 8:30 p.m. on one surgical floor, but with the quick success of the program, SJMH hopes to expand DART to all units in the hospital, and increase coverage to 16 hours per day.

The ADT at Grandview Hospital in Dayton, OH, is another pilot program designed to ease the burden of nurses and case managers and improve throughput, but its roots stem more from the ED. "We researched what bogged down our nurses the most and concluded [that] it was admissions," says **Greg Gibbons,** director of critical care at Grandview Hospital. "Getting a patient's history, performing an assessment, writing up a care plan based on problems—this can all take up to an hour or two based on the complexity of the case." And all of this work must occur while nurses continue to provide care for other patients in units and the ED.

Enter the ADT nurse. ADT nurses ease the burden of ED and floor nurses by facilitating the admission, assessment, and paperwork that go along with each patient, as well as providing ED-specific services to other areas of the hospital.

"Ideally, after an ADT nurse's work is done, a unit nurse would only have to do a report and a head-to-toe assessment," says Gibbons. "[He or she] essentially just [has] to put the patient in the bed and start from there."

In the ED, ADT nurses provide an extra level of care and support for patients, which has resulted in better throughput and fewer diversions. The ADT nurse expedites flow by providing aftercare to discharged patients and educating them and their families about prescribed treatments and medications and how and when to follow up with their primary care provider.

According to Gibbons, training an ADT team is easy if you have administration buy-in and qualified staff. All ADT nurses at Grandview were experienced ED nurses already familiar with doctors, staff, and patients. Similar to most ED teams, these nurses already possessed exceptional history-taking and assessment skills and were quite knowledgeable about coding and how to deal with complex, unstable patients. Therefore, ADT training and implementation focused more on scope over skills (i.e., how the program should run, its purpose and desired goals, etc.)

The ADT team determined that it could make the biggest impact by assisting all nurses with the arduous task of admissions and discharges. This is now the centerpiece of its mission.

When ADT was first introduced, other nurses throughout the hospital were skeptical. According to Gibbons, the general response was, "What exactly are they doing?" and "I wish I had a job like that." Gibbons reports that it took about a year before ADT caught on and nurses realized how much time it saved them.

"They really notice a difference now when an ADT nurse is not around," says Gibbons. "Now they say, 'Where is that ADT nurse, how come [he or she is] not around?' They've come to really appreciate that hour or so they save by having the ADT nurse do the admission and assessment."

Appreciation is widespread and nurse satisfaction has proven to be better than expected, reports Gibbons. ED and unit nurses trust ADT nurses and believe that the initial assessment and care that their patients receive from ADT nurses is excellent. Additionally, Grandview's length of stay, diversion rate, and incident reporting have all decreased.

"Every year when we do our budget review we evaluate what we can trim," says Gibbons. "We look at the ADT positions, and [decide that] these are not positions we're ever willing to slash. That's how valuable we feel they are."

Source: **Case Management Monthly,** HCPro, Inc., June 2006

Plan of care

About this facility

McKenzie-Willamette Medical Center, Springfield, OR

- 114 licensed beds
- Key services: adult/children's medicine, cardiac/neurology, cardiac cath, diagnostic imaging, emergency, endoscopy, general surgery, ICU, rehab, respiratory, women's health
- Last JCAHO survey: February 14, 2006

Plan of care

Why create a plan of care?

Many plans of care go unused and many nurses resent writing them—so why are they so important? Aside from the obvious benefit to the continuity of patient care, a nurse's license requires him or her to plan care for their patients. Most nurses are unaware that their board of nursing requires them, as part of patient care, to "develop and modify the plan of care for their patient."[1] Who knew? We knew that certain accrediting bodies, such as the Joint Commission on Accreditation of Healthcare Organizations (JCAHO), required a plan of care. Come to find out, it's also a requirement of a nurse's licensure. The Oregon State Board of Nursing defines a plan of care as

> *the written guidelines developed to identify specific problems of the individual and intervention/regimen necessary to assist individuals or groups to achieve optimal health potential. Developing the plan of care includes establishing client and nursing goals and determining nursing interventions to meet care objectives.*[2]

After looking at several nurse practice acts from several different states, I believe it's safe to say that we, as nurses, are required to initiate and update a plan of care for our patients. So as long as it is a requirement, why not make it a useful tool?

In 2001, I was assigned, along with a group of fellow nurses, the task of creating a care-delivery system at our hospital, McKenzie-Willamette Medical Center in Springfield, OR. We really had no idea what we were getting into. After almost two years we came up with processes and documentation tools that we hoped would make a safer care system. After five years, we have adapted, changed, and even given up on some of those tools and processes. But one tool/process that has stood the test of time and two JCAHO surveys was our plan of care. During our facility's last JCAHO survey, the plan of care was labeled a Best Practice.

Now that the "J" word has been mentioned, you may be surprised to know that you will not hear it again in this chapter. When our group got together we had some ground rules. One of those rules was to not quote JCAHO or Centers for Medicare & Medicaid Services standards. The idea was to create a safe care-delivery system. If we did this, we felt that we would achieve the necessary standards. As luck would have it, our finished product met all applicable standards.

In the following chapter I will describe to you what has made our care plan successful at our hospital. This is not to say that everything I mention will work in every hospital. The process for the care plan can be adjusted and "individualized" for each hospital. The bottom line is to deliver a plan of care that has value with frontline staff. If you take only one thing away from what you read here, know that this is the most important.

A brief history of the plan of care

Mention the word "Kardex" around most nurses these days, and you'll get a blank stare. The Kardex system faded out for the most part 15 to 20 years ago. In its day, it was a combination care plan, treatment reminder, and tool of communication about the patient. Many nurses considered it the "recipe card" for patient care (as a matter of fact, many Kardex systems used 5x7 note cards for documentation). By today's standard, this system seems antiquated, but it has two advantages over most of our modern systems: easy access and patient-specific information.

For most, our first negative experience with the plan of care was in nursing school. This set the stage for most nurses to dislike—and maybe even fear—the plan of care. It was not uncommon in nursing school to write pages and pages of care plans. Throw in nursing diagnoses, a few "related tos" and "associated withs," and the next thing you knew you had a monster of a care plan that only your nursing instructor would have time to read through. How could this be used as a communication tool in the real world if it took 20 minutes to read and digest information on just one patient? What we didn't know as students was that for the most part, the plan of care was used as an educational tool to measure what the student had learned. The care plan illustrated the student's thought process and understanding of the disease process.

 Nursing Assessment, Plan of Care, and Patient Education: The Foundation of Patient Care

Finally we became employed as real, licensed, registered nurses. Along with our fresh, "change-the-world" attitude, we brought our advanced know-how on how to write a complete and comprehensive 12-page care plan. We quickly learned that when caring for six patients at the same time, you didn't have the time to write a detailed plan of care for every issue affecting your patient. "Hit the high points," many new nurses were told. Then, for many of us, came the comment, "Besides, no one looks at the care plan anyway."

Most nurses work with one of two types of care plans, either handwritten or computer generated. As most hospitals continue to move to the electronic medical record and point-of-care documentation, the handwritten plan of care is becoming less and less common. Both formats have their advantages and disadvantages, which we will discuss later.

As the plan of care has continued to evolve over time, the addition of other disciplines' information to the plan of care has resulted in the multidisciplinary plan of care. This addition has resulted in two notable changes. First, the plan of care has become much broader in scope, therefore becoming more useful. The second notable change is that other disciplines, such as respiratory therapy, speech therapy, occupational therapy, physical therapy, care management, even dietary, update the plan of care. It is amazing how many other hospitals I have spoken with who state that their care plan is poorly updated by nursing, "but the therapies use it all the time."

Why the plan of care fails

The top reasons cited for why the plan of care fails are:

- It's too generic
- There's too much information
- It isn't part of the normal work flow
- I have too many other places to document
- I don't update it because no one reads it
- I don't read it because no one updates it
- I don't have the time

In many instances, the reasons listed above are valid from the staff nurse's perspective. The care plan has to be viewed as a valuable tool that can easily be accessed and is helpful to the patient. Instead, many nurses view the plan of care as busy work.

Generic care plans

If a care plan is generic, which many are, the nurse is guaranteed that no one will use it. Whether you are currently using a computerized documentation system, or are still using paper, generic care plans can be found in both systems. You can easily spot generic care plans when you take two patients' plans (with similar diagnosis) and set them side by side. In reading through them you see no (or very few) differences between the plans. In order to be useful, the plan has to be individualized for each patient.

For example, even though Mr. Smith and Mr. Jones both have congestive heart failure, Mr. Smith has new-onset diabetes, and Mr. Jones has chronic obstructive pulmonary disease (COPD). They both share the same primary diagnosis, but their treatments, and therefore their care plans, should have many differences. Also keep in mind that the care plan should be prioritized. This helps individualize the care plan, as well as focus other staff working with the patient on what may be the most important issues at which to look.

In hospitals that are using computerized documentation, the care plan is usually generated from a list of available, diagnosis-related problems. It is not uncommon to see the same problem chosen for all patients that share the same diagnosis. Some systems allow a certain degree of individualization of the problem, but unfortunately, this is rarely utilized. Many systems allow only the basic problem, solution, and outcome. This creates a very generic care plan with very little value to the staff nurse.

Some hospitals are still writing care plans by hand. In my opinion, these are the care plans that have the most hope for individualization. Unfortunately, when these care plans are written, the nurse usually draws from a list of common problems, solutions, and outcomes he or she has developed over years of writing care plans. It is the human equivalent of the computerized documentation system.

The flip side of the generic care plan is the "telephone book." This huge care plan is designed to baffle you with so much information that you don't even try to read it. This is similar to the plans of care nurses completed as students. The funny thing about it is that it is still very generic. The author usually has a standard set of problems and outcomes for a specific diagnosis. The problems are so buried in anatomy, physiology, and the disease process, that it goes unread due to its sheer size. Unless a patient has been on your floor for quite a while, you shouldn't be seeing a five- or six-page care plan. Imagine for a moment needing to update this monstrous plan of care. This is not a user-friendly care plan and therefore will not be utilized.

Other factors that can cause a care plan's failure

There are a few environmental factors that may affect the use of the care plan. Are there enough computer terminals? Is the written plan of care located in an area that is easily accessible? Is the care plan part of the nurse's usual work flow? At our hospital, we had a paper documentation system, with one exception: the care plan. A nurse had to log in to the computer, and then create or update the plan of care. We were asking our nurses to do everything in one system EXCEPT the plan of care. What priority do you think the plan of care received?

Probably the most common reason the care plan fails is the lack of importance the bedside nurse places in it. As mentioned previously, many nurses view the care plan as busy work. Staff nurses don't have time to waste, so if they view something as unnecessary, it will not be completed. How many times has a staff nurse uttered, "I don't update the care plan, because no one reads it."? The next nurse says, "I don't read the care plan, because no one ever updates it." This is what I call the "Vicious Cycle of the Plan of Care." The plan of care has to be an integral part of the nurse's day. It needs to be filled with information that the nurse finds valuable.

Goals of the new care plan

When my group began to think of ways to create a safe care-delivery system, one of the main areas of improvement we focused on was the continuity of care for our patients. A recurring problem on the floors was that vital information was lost between shifts. It seemed as though each nurse was only able to see his or her eight-hour shift, and couldn't look forward or back. This was a problem with today's severely acute patients. We wondered, what were we missing in the report? What were we missing in our nursing documentation? Where was the continuity of care?

When our group looked deeper into our documentation, we found that the information was being adequately recorded (keep in mind, this was a paper record). The problem was accessing the information after it was documented. If you were the oncoming nurse, you might need to scan through a page of narrative documentation to see what happened in the last 24 hours. If you had to look back over the last few days, you were in real trouble.

With our previous system, a written report was completed for the next shift. There was also time between shifts for the oncoming and off-going shifts to touch base. But for the most part, the information from report was not making it past the eight hours of the next shift. When we began using the care plan model that I will describe later, we began seeing a notable decrease in missed items on subsequent shifts. Our care plan turned into a multidisciplinary, ongoing report tool. By providing a place to document ongoing patient issues in a concise, easy-to-read format, the care plan can noticeably increase the continuity of patient care.

Elements of a successful care plan

To create a successful care plan, we decided that our new plan would have to be everything our old plan wasn't. Our new plan of care had to be

1. useful to staff
2. easy to access and update
3. patient specific
4. multidisciplinary

It would seem that these elements are obvious, but as we researched the tools other hospitals were using, we found that we were all in the same boat. So if most people understood what the care plan should be, why were so many hospitals having trouble making their care plan a success? In my opinion, your care plan will never succeed (or at least reach its full potential), until you have buy-in from staff. The staff nurse will see zero value in the plan of care if it does not help him or her to care for the patient.

To help make your plan more accessible and useful to staff nurses, ask yourself the following questions:

- If the system you use is still based in paper (as was ours), or you document electronically, what does the staff nurse (and for that matter any other discipline) have to go through to initiate and update the plan of care? Do they have to search for the plan of care?

- Are there enough computer terminals for easy access to the plan of care?

- Once they have the plan of care, is it easy to access?

- Is the plan of care something that is in their normal work flow?

Any one of the issues above can cause the plan of care to fail.

To ensure that your developing plan will be an individualized, meaningful plan, ask yourself and your team, "Does the care plan speak about a particular patient, or does it just look at a diagnosis?" If the care plan is generic, it will not be useful to staff.

To help make your plan more individualized, ask the following questions:

- Start by looking at the patient. What is the history that brought this patient to the hospital?

- Aside from his or her admitting diagnosis, what else is keeping this patient from attaining his or her highest possible level of wellness?

- What are we currently doing for the patient?

Lastly, in order to make the plan of care truly successful, you need to lose the idea of the "nursing plan of care." If you haven't already, you need to get buy-in from all the other disciplines. When your care plan is multidisciplinary, it becomes even more individualized, and much more useful to the staff using it. Imagine having the opportunity to scan through easy-to-read documents that focus on the patient's needs from the perspectives of all disciplines caring for the patient. Many times as nurses, we wonder who else is seeing the patient and what progress is being made. In many systems, this is accomplished by looking through the medical record under several different sections, or even more commonly, chasing down a therapist in the hallway to compare notes on the patient's prognosis. This information can be more accessible in a multidisciplinary plan of care.

The final product

After working on and refining care plans for more than two years, our group was amazed at how simple our final product was. But, we've found our care plan's simplicity is what makes it work so well. Keep in mind, I will be taking you through the process that worked at our hospital. There is probably no way to implement this complete process in another hospital. What you will learn are the factors that helped us make a useful care plan.

Previously we documented everything on paper except the plan of care. We had tried over the years to make this computerized "canned" plan of care easier. We got to the point where the problems and outcomes were completely blank, forcing the staff nurse to enter text every time he or she created the care plan. This was actually successful in getting the initial or admission plan of care entered in the computer, and then placed in the chart. However, at discharge, you would find the same care plan, rarely added to, almost never updated, sitting in the chart. Other disciplines had no real reason to enter data into the computer either. We wound up with a nursing-focused care plan that showed the patient at admission.

We kept the majority of current information regarding the patient at a bedside nurse server, such as the nurse's notes and patient education tool. Most of the information that the RN needed to access was at the bedside—even the plan of care. The obvious problem was that the nurse had to walk past the care plan, down the hall, and find a computer to update the plan. Even after we installed a number of new computer terminals, the plan of care was not being updated (and therefore not being used). The only reason the nurse had to login into the computer was to update the plan of care. This was a significant deviation from the nurse's usual work flow, and therefore it failed.

Our only option was to make our bedside documentation handwritten. In an age of PCs, cell phones, and PDAs, we opted to take a step back in history, and return to pen and paper. I won't say that this gave us the perfect care plan overnight, but an immediate change occurred. Suddenly all the staff caring for the patient could walk into a patient's room and access and update the care plan. The plan of care was now in a location that the nurse and other disciplines frequented with every visit to the patient.

The basic form we used for our care plan can be found in Figure 2.1 and Figure 2.2. After discussing our wants and needs with our information technology department, they produced this basic form. We asked them to pull out as much useful information from our computer system, and have it automatically print on the form to be used. If you look at Section A on Figure 2.1, you will see that with our current system we were able to get patient name, room number, age, account number, medical record number, physician name, publicity code, allg, code status, isolation precautions' and admit date.

During the admission process, our nurses usually log into a computer. Since they are already on the computer, any information they put in at this point is naturally part of their work flow. This brings us to Section B of Figure 2.1. Our nurses type a brief medical history of the patient including prior health issues, prior hospitalizations, and a brief history of recent issues that led them to be admitted to the hospital. I have received feedback that this is one of the most useful parts of the care plan. A patient can be in the hospital for less than 24 hours and any discipline walking into the room can get a brief history on the patient.

In looking at Section C of Figure 2.1, you see the area for department consults. As with most hospitals, we have set criteria for when a patient should be referred to another department. During admission, any necessary department referrals are placed in the computer as an order. The system then draws that information over to the care plan so it's on the sheet when it's printed. Several times, I have heard nurses at hospitals complain that it is not always easy to find what departments have been referred.

Once the patient history and department referrals have been entered, the care plan is printed, and is now that patient's basic plan of care. The nurse will never need to go back to the computer again to update the care plan. At this point, the care plan appears as Figure 2.1 and Figure 2.2. Figure 2.2 is simply the format for the second and subsequent pages. At our hospital we automatically print a second page to make it easy to access and use.

The care plan can now be written on by the admitting nurse and subsequent staff nurses caring for the patient. To make the care plan useful and easy to use, we decided that we needed to know two things: What is wrong with the patient, and how we are going to fix it. With that in mind, we made a problem column, action column, and goal column. The rule was to write the problem, action, and goal in plain English. Avoid long sentences and "medicalese" as much as possible. Looking at Figure 2.3, you see the patient's first problem was sinus tachycardia. The action we took was IV hydration and having the patient on a cardiac monitor. The goal was a return to normal sinus rhythm (NSR). Incredibly simple, and incredibly easy to write, update, and access.

On the care plan you will also see a start-date column. This column is used for two purposes. The nurse enters the date he or she entered the problem on the care plan, and he or she also enters his or her initials. Our hospital only requires initials instead of a signature. We have initiated a signature sheet that we keep on the chart. Any person caring for a particular patient writes their initials, title, printed name and signature. This makes documentation simpler—you only need to place your initials on any form you use in the medical record as long as you have entered the appropriate information on the signature sheet.

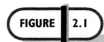

Plan of care

Sat. Oct. 8, 2005 08:26   MWMC Plan of Care Pg. 1

10/8/05 Shift 1 through 10/8/05 Shift 3

SECTION A

ACM 20-D WITT, FRED	41Y ACCT#:052356661 MR#:UNIT3
BARNHART, RICHARD PUB:	Dx: 786.6-CHEST SWELLING
Allg:	Code: Iso:
Precautions:	ADM DATE: 10/8/05

SECTION B

PATIENT HISTORY

Peripheral neuropathy, CHF, hypertension, chronic peripheral edema, aortic stenosis, A-fib, anemia, pneumonia, new dx of adenocarcinoma
Obesity, ruptured gall bladder, type-2 diabetic, currently insulin dependent, severe osteoarthritis, lumbar comp fx. Increased SOB, fever/chills, increased chest discomfort x4 days.

SECTION C

DEPARTMENT CONSULTS
50   CNS CHAPLAINCY- CONSULTS   10/10/05 09:22   ROUTINE
Please visit pt

CONSULTS DATE	DPT	REASON	INITIAL CONTACT DATE/TIME/SIGNATURE	ORDER#

SECTION D

START DATE	DPT	PROBLEM	ACTION	GOAL	STOP DATE	PRIORITY

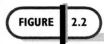

Plan of care

Sat. Oct. 8, 2005 08:26   MWMC Plan of Care Pg. 2

10/8/05 Shift 1 through 10/8/05 Shift 3

ACM 20-D   WITT, FRED   41Y   ACCT#:052356661   MR#: UNIT#
BARNHART, RICHARD   PUB: Dx: 786.6-CHEST SWELLING
Allg: Code: Iso:
Precautions: ADM DATE: 10/8/05

START DATE	DPT	PROBLEM	ACTION	GOAL	STOP DATE	PRIORITY

The department column is an easy way to determine which discipline has entered the problem. In our hospital, the following departments/disciplines enter information on the plan of care:

- Nursing
- Pharmacy
- Physical, Occupational, and Speech Therapy
- Respiratory therapy
- Enterostomal therapy
- Care management
- Infection control
- Chaplaincy

This creates a truly multidisciplinary, informative care plan. It allows the care plan to show the patient in a holistic manner.

Next, look at the priority column of Figure 2.3. Many hospitals try to numerically prioritize the care of a patient. If you have more than eight problems, it becomes difficult to determine what should be number one and number two (sometimes it's obvious, but in most cases, several problems may seem appropriate for first and second priority). Our group decided not to prioritize numerically, but to divide all problems into three levels: high, medium, and low. We then looked at the average length of stay on the medical floor, 3.14 days. We decided that nursing and other disciplines would not have adequate time to address any low-priority issues. Based on this, we decided to prioritize problems as either medium or high. That is not to say a lower-priority problem could not eventually make it onto the care plan, it only meant that at the point it did, we had already addressed every other medium- and high-priority problem already on the plan of care. Now the nurse only had to focus on two priorities for the plan of care.

Now look at Figure 2.4. The patient's original problem was lower back pain. The action was to give pain medications with a goal of decreased pain. For the purposes of this example, we'll say that this problem was originally written on the night shift. By the evening shift, the nurse caring for the patient has a pretty good idea that Vicodin can be used to control the patient's pain. At this point the nurse completes the goal by writing the stop date in the stop date column, and using a highlighter to yellow the problem out. The nurse can then write a revised problem. Look at Figure 2.5. You can see that the nurse has written the problem again, but it is now more specific with the

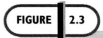

Plan of care

| Sat. Oct. 8, 2005 08:26 | | | MWMC Plan of Care Pg. 1 | | | |

10/8/05 Shift 1 through 10/8/05 Shift 3

SECTION A

ACM 20-D WITT, FRED	41Y ACCT#:052356661 MR#:UNIT3
BARNHART, RICHARD PUB:	Dx: 786.6-CHEST SWELLING
Allg:	Code: Iso:
Precautions:	ADM DATE: 10/8/05

SECTION B

PATIENT HISTORY

Peripheral neuropathy, CHF, hypertension, chronic peripheral edema, aortic stenosis, A-fib, anemia, pneumonia, new dx of adenocarcinoma

Obesity, ruptured gall bladder, type-2 diabetic, currently insulin dependent, severe osteoarthritis, lumbar comp fx. Increased SOB, fever/chills, increased chest discomfort x4 days.

SECTION C

DEPARTMENT CONSULTS

50   CNS CHAPLAINCY- CONSULTS   10/8/05   09:22   ROUTINE

Please visit pt

CONSULTS DATE	DPT	REASON	INITIAL CONTACT DATE/TIME/SIGNATURE	ORDER#

SECTION D

START DATE	DPT	PROBLEM	ACTION	GOAL	STOP DATE	PRIORITY
10/8/05	NSG	Sinus tach	IV hydration monitor	Return to NSR		H
10/8/05	NSG	Pneumonia w/resp. distress	Sat O2, monitor resp. status, monitor for sepsis	Resolve		H
10/8/05	NSG	Chronic low back pain	Monitor pain, offer pain meds	↓ lwr back pain		M
10/8/05	NSG	DX of CA, Depression	Offer emotional support, consult for chaplain	Chaplain to see Pt.		H
10/8/05	NSG	Chronic Periph Edema	Monitor for ↑ edema-MED w/diuretic as ordered	Edema @ baseline		M

action. Now any nurse looking at this plan of care can see that Vicodin is working to control the patient's pain. You can also see that the nurse has revised the problem regarding peripheral edema. Specific orders for diuretics are now documented, as well as a priority change from medium to high. Also note that respiratory therapy has become involved and added a problem involving shortness of breath.

Continuing through the plan of care in chronological order, now look at Figure 2.6. For the purpose of demonstrating the flow of the plan of care, we'll say the patient has been in the hospital for 24 hours, and it is now October 9. The first thing you will notice is documentation in Section C of the care plan. As previously mentioned, our hospital puts department referrals in as an order in the computer system. When they are entered at admit, they appear on the plan of care automatically. With Mr. Witt, the patient on the plan of care, the nurse decided that he has probable home-care issues. The nurse has written the problem related to the home-care issue, and has had a consult placed in the computer system. The nurse then writes on the plan of care, under the referral section (Section C), the date of the referral, the department referred, and a brief reason why the patient was referred. At this point, any other staff member looking at this care plan will know that this particular issue is being addressed. Also note on Figure 2.7 that the chaplain has addressed the issue she was consulted for at admission.

Moving on to Figure 2.8, it is now October 10. In the referral area C, you will see when the care manager saw the patient. She also entered a problem on the plan of care (Figure 2.9), and discontinued the previous problem nursing had originally entered. Again, being able to follow the referral process from start to finish has been confusing at times. Area C is a place to refer, to see if a referral was made, why the referral was made, and the referred department's follow up. This alone has been a significant time saver for nurses and other disciplines.

Another example of how the care plan can help facilitate continuity of care can be found in the case of an elderly patient who is admitted to the medical floor through the emergency department in the late evening. As part of the admission process, the nurse asks the patient if she has had her pnuemoccocal vaccine. The patient responds with, "I can't remember." At this point, the scenario can go two different ways. The nurse can write in her report for the oncoming shifts to ask the physician when he rounds tomorrow, and hope the message makes it through to shift. What is more likely to happen is that the ball will be dropped, and it won't be addressed until discharge. The discharge process is a bottleneck already, as you are trying to complete every last-minute thing to get the patient safely out

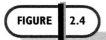

FIGURE 2.4

Plan of care

Sat. Oct. 8, 2005 08:26   MWMC Plan of Care Pg. 1

10/8/05 Shift 1 through 10/8/05 Shift 3

SECTION A

ACM 20-D WITT, FRED	41Y ACCT#:052356661 MR#:UNIT3
BARNHART, RICHARD PUB:	Dx: 786.6-CHEST SWELLING
Allg:	Code: Iso:
Precautions:	ADM DATE: 10/8/05

SECTION B

PATIENT HISTORY

Peripheral neuropathy, CHF, hypertension, chronic peripheral edema, aortic stenosis, A-fib, anemia, pneumonia, new dx of adenocarcinoma
Obesity, ruptured gall bladder, type-2 diabetic, currently insulin dependent, severe osteoarthritis, lumbar comp fx. Increased SOB, fever/chills, increased chest discomfort x4 days.

SECTION C

DEPARTMENT CONSULTS
50   CNS CHAPLAINCY- CONSULTS   10/10/05 09:22   ROUTINE
Please visit pt

CONSULTS DATE	DPT	REASON	INITIAL CONTACT DATE/TIME/SIGNATURE	ORDER#

SECTION D

START DATE	DPT	PROBLEM	ACTION	GOAL	STOP DATE	PRIORITY
10/8/05	NSG	Sinus tach	IU hydration monitor	Return to NSR		H
10/8/05	NSG	Pneumonia w/resp. distress	Sat O2, monitor resp. status, monitor for sepsis	Resolve		H
10/8/05	NSG	Chronic low back pain	Monitor pain, offer pain meds	↓ lwr back pain	10/8/05	M
10/8/05	NSG	DX of CA, Depression	Offer emotional support, consult for chaplain	Chaplain to see Pt.		H
10/8/05	NSG	Chronic Periph Edema	Monitor for edema-MED w/diuretic as ordered	Edema @ baseline	10/8/05	M

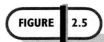

Plan of care

Sat. Oct. 8, 2005 08:26   MWMC Plan of Care Pg. 2

10/8/05 Shift 1 through 10/8/05 Shift 3

ACM 20-D   WITT, FRED   41Y   ACCT#:052356661   MR#:UNIT3
BARNHART, RICHARD   PUB: Dx: 786.6-CHEST SWELLING
Allg: Code: Iso:
Precautions: ADM DATE: 10/8/05

START DATE	DPT	PROBLEM	ACTION	GOAL	STOP DATE	PRIORITY
10/8/05	NSG	Lower back pain	2 vicodin every 4 hrs. to relieve	↓ back pain		M
10/8/05	NSG	Periph Edema	Lasix ↑ to 40 mg. T.I.D. watch K+	Edema @baseline		H
10/8/05	RT	SOB, ↑ O2 needs	Aerosol Tx adjust O2 to Protocol	To room air		H

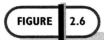

Plan of care

Sun. Oct. 9, 2005 08:26   MWMC Plan of Care Pg. 1

10/9/05 Shift 1 through 10/9/05 Shift 3

SECTION A

ACM 20-D WITT, FRED	41Y ACCT#:052356661 MR#:UNIT3
BARNHART, RICHARD PUB:	Dx: 786.6-CHEST SWELLING
Allg:	Code: Iso:
Precautions:	ADM DATE: 10/8/05

SECTION B

PATIENT HISTORY

Peripheral neuropathy, CHF, hypertension, chronic peripheral edema, aortic stenosis, A-fib, anemia, pneumonia, new dx of adenocarcinoma
Obesity, ruptured gall bladder, type-2 diabetic, currently insulin dependent, severe osteoarthritis, lumbar comp fx. Increased SOB, fever/chills, increased chest discomfort x4 days.

SECTION C

DEPARTMENT CONSULTS
50   CNS CHAPLAINCY- CONSULTS   10/10/05 09:22   ROUTINE
Please visit pt

CONSULTS DATE	DPT	REASON	INITIAL CONTACT DATE/TIME/SIGNATURE	ORDER#
10/9/05	CM	Home care issues		#81

SECTION D

START DATE	DPT	PROBLEM	ACTION	GOAL	STOP DATE	PRIORITY
10/8/05	NSG	Sinus tach	IU hydration monitor	Return to NSR		H
10/8/05	NSG	Pneumonia w/resp. distress	Sat O2, monitor resp. status, monitor for sepsis	Resolve		H
10/8/05	NSG	Chronic low back pain	Monitor pain, offer pain meds	↓ lwr back pain	10/8/05	M
10/8/05	NSG	DX of CA, Depression	Offer emotional support, consult for chaplain	Chaplain to see Pt.		H
10/8/05	NSG	Chronic Periph Edema	Monitor for edema- MED w/diuretic as ordered	Edema @ baseline	10/8/05	M

the door. The other scenario has the admitting nurse writing a problem in the care plan: "Patient unsure of pneumovax status." Action: "Speak with MD in morning." Goal: "Clarify status."

As the care plan is updated, new problems are added and some are completed. If the care plan were to get into multiple pages, the nurse can easily skim through the problem list, ignoring the yellowed-out problems that have been discontinued. If she is looking for a more in-depth picture of the patient, she can read through the care plan, looking at both current as well as discontinued problems to get a better idea of the patient's hospital course.

Our care plan was successful. By successful, I mean we were seeing about a 60%–70% compliance rate with our care plan. It was being updated, prioritized and it actually gave you current, relevant information on the patient. Then the group met again. What could we do to increase nurses' compliance with using the tool? What is the most important thing that the nurse uses to plan their workday? What one item, if taken away, would cause the nurse to come to a screeching halt until he or she recovered it? The answer is the report sheet.

Shift-to-shift report is done many different ways at many different hospitals. What if the care plan, and other supporting documentation that the nurse uses every day could be put together to create an intershift report tool? The more we thought about it, the more we liked it. We weren't asking the nurses to do more work—they were already writing on a report sheet every shift—we were just asking them to write the information in a different place.

We decided to put together a folder of information that remains at the bedside. It contains the documentation tools and information needed to care for the patient. The folder contains

- nursing admission assessment (a more complete history than on the care plan)
- fall-risk assessment (completed every shift, shows history of fall risk)
- signature/initial form
- care plan
- nurses' notes
- patient education tool (what the patient knows, and what needs reinforcement)
- discharge teaching tool (it's never too early to start)

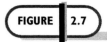

Plan of care

Sun. Oct. 9, 2005 08:26   MWMC Plan of Care Pg. 2

10/9/05 Shift 1 through 10/9/05 Shift 3

ACM 20-D   WITT, FRED   41Y   ACCT#:052356661   MR#:UNIT3
BARNHART, RICHARD   PUB: Dx: 786.6-CHEST SWELLING
Allg: Code: Iso:
Precautions: ADM DATE: 10/8/05

START DATE	DPT	PROBLEM	ACTION	GOAL	STOP DATE	PRIORITY
10/8/05	NSG	Lower back pain	2 vicodin every 4 hrs. to relieve	↓ back pain		M
10/8/05	NSG	Periph Edema	Lasix to 40 mg. T.I.D. watch K+	Edema @baseline		H
10/8/05	RT	SOB, ↑ O2 needs	Aerosol Tx adjust O2 to Protocol	To room air		H
10/8/05	Chapln	New Dx of CA	Spoke w/patient, gave emotional support, will cont. w/F/U visits during pt's stay	Provide support		H
10/9/05	NSG	Pt. states he and sister are only caregivers to elderly mother. Sister has stolen money in the past	Consult CM to see if social services can get involved	CM consult		H

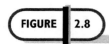 **Plan of care**

| Mon. Oct. 10, 2005 08:26 | | | | MWMC Plan of Care Pg. 1 | | |

10/10/05 Shift 1 through 10/10/05 Shift 3

SECTION A

ACM 20-D WITT, FRED			41Y ACCT#:052356661 MR#:UNIT3
BARNHART, RICHARD PUB:			Dx: 786.6-CHEST SWELLING
Allg:			Code: Iso:
Precautions:			ADM DATE: 10/8/05

SECTION B

PATIENT HISTORY

Peripheral neuropathy, CHF, hypertension, chronic peripheral edema, aortic stenosis, A-fib, anemia, pneumonia, new dx of adenocarcinoma

Obesity, ruptured gall bladder, type-2 diabetic, currently insulin dependent, severe osteoarthritis, lumbar comp fx. Increased SOB, fever/chills, increased chest discomfort x4 days.

SECTION C

DEPARTMENT CONSULTS

50   CNS CHAPLAINCY- CONSULTS   10/10/05 09:22   ROUTINE
Please visit pt

CONSULTS DATE	DPT	REASON	INITIAL CONTACT DATE/TIME/SIGNATURE	ORDER#
10/9/05	CM	Home care issues	10/10/05/0930 L.Bar C.M	#81

SECTION D

START DATE	DPT	PROBLEM	ACTION	GOAL	STOP DATE	PRIORITY
10/8/05	NSG	Sinus tach	IU hydration monitor	Return to NSR		H
10/8/05	NSG	Pneumonia w/resp. distress	Sat O2, monitor resp. status, monitor for sepsis	Resolve		H
10/8/05	NSG	Chronic low back pain	Monitor pain, offer pain meds	▼ lwr back pain	10/8/05	M
10/8/05	NSG	DX of CA, Depression	Offer emotional support, consult for chaplain	Chaplain to see Pt.		H
10/8/05	NSG	Chronic Periph Edema	Monitor for edema- MED w/diuretic as ordered	Edema @ baseline	10/8/05	M

 ©2006 HCPro, Inc.   Nursing Assessment, Plan of Care, and Patient Education: The Foundation of Patient Care

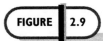 **FIGURE 2.9**

Plan of care

Mon. Oct. 10, 2005 08:26   MWMC Plan of Care Pg. 2

10/10/05 Shift 1 through 10/10/05 Shift 3

ACM 20-D   WITT, FRED   41Y   ACCT#:052356661   MR#:UNIT3
BARNHART, RICHARD   PUB: Dx: 786.6-CHEST SWELLING
Allg: Code: Iso:
Precautions: ADM DATE: 10/8/05

START DATE	DPT	PROBLEM	ACTION	GOAL	STOP DATE	PRIORITY
10/8/05	NSG	Lower back pain	2 vicodin every 4 hrs. to relieve	↓ back pain		M
10/8/05	NSG	Periph Edema	Lasix ↑ to 40 mg. T.I.D. watch K+	Edema @baseline		H
10/8/05	RT	SOB, ↑ O2 needs	Aerosol Tx adjust O2 to Protocol	To room air		H
10/8/05	Chapln	New Dx of CA	Spoke w/patient, gave emotional support, will cont. w/F/U visits during pt's stay	Provide support		H
10/9/05	NSG	Pt. states he and sister are only caregivers to elderly mother. Sister has stolen money in the past	Consult CM to see if social services can get involved	CM consult	10/10/05	H
10/10/05	NSG	Pt's sister came into Pt room, verbally abusive. Sister escorted from hospital	Security alert placed	Sister will not return		H
10/10/05	CM	F/U w/ pt. concern, re: mother's care	F/U w/ social worker to send case worker to mother's house	Patient feels safe w/mother's living arrangement		H

This folder may seem to contain a significant amount of information, but keep in mind that this is how the oncoming nurse will get his or her report. If there is an issue that will last well into the next shift and/or beyond, it goes on the care plan. If it is something that is short term and the oncoming nurse needs to know right away, it is verbalized in our inter-shift hand-off communication. Also know that every form has a specific place within the folder. You know what page the care plan is on every time. You can also go to any inpatient unit and find the bedside folder in the same order. Your float staff will be very pleased.

Now that the care plan has become part of the report process, it is updated every shift as needed. A surveyor at our facility coined an interesting phrase to describe what we developed, "A living, breathing document of the patient's planned care." The more I thought about it, the more I agreed with her. You can pick up the care plan of one of our patients and get individualized, up-to-date information on that patient.

Adapting the care plan to meet your needs

This information is meant to help you define, at your hospital, how you could improve your care-planning process. In order for it to work for your facility, you must individualize (much like the care plan itself) some of the concepts I have mentioned. Some facilities have completely gone electronic. Can the concepts I have mentioned help in these facilities? Absolutely. As the word from surveyors has gotten out over the last year, I get at least one call or e-mail a week asking for more information on this "Best Practice" care plan. When I send the information, and then follow up on the phone, people seem a little puzzled. I can tell they are thinking, "This is it?" The overall process is very simple; perhaps this is what has prevented people from doing it in the past. In the age of computers, to handwrite something on a nearly blank sheet of paper seems like we are stepping back into the Stone Age. I have gotten over that. If it works, use it.

As you begin to advance your plan of care, keep some of these simple, but important thoughts in mind:

- Invite staff nurses to be on the committee that will revise the care plan. They are on the floor every day. Their insight is invaluable.

- Make sure the care plan is viewed as a useful tool. Is it something the staff nurse seeks out?

- Make the care plan part of the normal workflow.

- Make it easy to use. That means it's easily accessible and easy to update. Problems, actions, and outcomes should be short and concise.

- Train any discipline that cares for the patient on how to update the care plan.

- Try prioritizing in a simple manner. You can try just using medium and high. You can also just prioritize the top six problems. A staff nurse is not realistically going to get past the top six problems in his or her shift.

- And lastly, make it simple.

References:

1 Oregon State Board of Nursing, *Nurse Practice Act,* Division 45
2 Oregon Board of Nursing, *Nurse Practice Act,,* 851-045-0000, (3), (m)

Case Study #3: Documentation system coordinates assessments and care plans

Shawnee Mission (KS) Medical Center had a successful Joint Commission on Accrediatation of Healthcare Organizations (JCAHO) survey, partly due to their documentation system designed to compel staff to work together and consistently coordinate patients' care plans.

The facility's documentation forms streamline the following four elements of documentation for all departments to create multidisciplinary charting:

- Admission assessment
- Physical assessment findings
- Plan of care and path
- Discharge education

Each of the four areas has its own separate form.

The forms help busy staff members prioritize patients' treatment plans from admission through discharge, says **Susan Stark, RN, MSN, CS, ARNP,** Shawnee Mission's neuro-clinical nurse specialist.

The forms also make it easier for staff to visualize and document the patient's care process, like fitting pieces of a puzzle together.

"The JCAHO liked the way we connected our documentation," Stark says. "It helped us with the survey since we could articulate the patient care processes well, which is really important."

Simplification and consistency

About four years ago, Shawnee Mission leaders decided to make it easier for nurses to track all of the required assessment screens that range from nutritional screens to the history and physical exams.

Leaders also wanted to create a policy to "document by exception," meaning nurses should focus on describing abnormal assessments and responses.

This proved to be a challenge because nurses vary greatly in how they describe an assessment or a response, Stark says. The hospital also wanted to clearly define care standards so that caregivers document consistently.

"By clearly defining assessment parameters, nurses could check a box stating a patient meets the defined assessment," she says.

The forms offer multiple descriptors by body system to allow nurses to describe the patient variations from the defined assessment. "Nurses must consistently document assessment parameters to communicate changes in patient condition and alterations in the plan of care to support these changes," Stark says.

Ensuring timely referrals

The forms link a patient's past medical history and current health problem, with a "problem priority" column that runs along the right hand side of the template. The problem column prompts nurses to note, for example, if they discover a gastrointestinal (GI) problem when filling out the GI section.

This process ensures that caregivers note a problem and alert the appropriate department (e.g., notifying occupational therapy if nursing checks off "slurred speech").

In another example, if nursing notes a problem while filling in the dietary screen, they will call in the dietary staff for referrals. Or, if a patient has complex wounds, staff can consult the wound-care center clinicians.

"We guide patient care throughout the hospitalization with the personal problem list," Stark says. And, if a new problem arises—such as forming pressure ulcers during the hospital stay—nurses can modify the outcomes and plan of care by adding interventions.

The hospital also wanted to tie in patient outcome improvement projects, such as reducing patient falls. So staff devoted one section to fall-risk assessments, and developed a fall-risk reduction protocol, Stark says.

Collaborating on screening

Ensuring appropriate discharge planning upon admission is also important—and a standard requirement. The forms incorporate interdepartmental staff planning in this area, too. For example, social workers helped to develop the continuum-of-care portion of the screen, which deals with discharge planning, Stark says.

Staff consult social workers to assist with the problems identified in this section at admission. Perhaps the patient will need a home health aide, which staff realize upon completing the screen. "The screen drives staff to think about what they can accomplish and plan for before the patient goes home," she says.

The challenge with multidisciplinary charting is getting staff members to think differently about documentation, Stark says.

It's not easy to get staff to document and plan together when they are used to doing it alone. However, working together shortens the time spent planning and documenting, thus reducing patients' length of stay in the long run.

United project

Creating the forms entailed staff input. "We wanted to have our documentation developed by our clinical experts," Stark says. "We wanted our clinical staff to have a final decision on what the tool looks like." This was crucial, because these are the people who use it, she says.

Shawnee Mission piloted the forms for a few months before using them to smooth out any glitches and to get staff feedback.

"Even the physicians bought into this," she says. "We found that they use the data that nurses gather from patients and that this form is easier to read. Physicians find it's a better way to check on nuances in the data when treating patients." Patients have better care coordination during their stay

because they know that all caregivers are on the same page—or same form—and everyone has the same information.

Redefining processes

When Shawnee Mission first started to work on the forms, they focused primarily on improving documentation.

But staff quickly realized they needed to go back and define the hospital's practices so that the document supports what they do. "So, if anyone else out there plans to have a similar project, we'd like to save them from making our mistake, which was starting backwards," Stark says.

Staff rebuilt their patient-care standards to ensure they fit the documentation format, which, they say, took more time.

Source: **Briefings on JCAHO,** May 2002, HCPro, Inc.

Case Study #4: Hand-off communication and care plans

One facility ties a plan of care document to the process

Hand-off communication goes beyond the shift-to-shift, nurse-to-nurse report, according to clinical interdisciplinary team managers at Youville Hospital & Rehabilitation Center in Cambridge, MA.

These managers developed a form to help them comply not only with the JCAHO's 2006 National Patient Safety Goal for hand-off communication, but to follow-up on all of their patients' initial plans of care.

"It's our ongoing hand-off for everybody," says Janet Hosta, RN, MSN, director of professional development at Youville. "We consider it to be a hand-off because it's in the record and it's reviewed by anybody taking care of the patient."

Addressing a problem

When patients are admitted to Youville, staff fill out a six-page initial interdisciplinary care form that individualizes a patient's plan of care.

The problem was that the form wasn't revisited, Hosta says.

"We were not going back to the original care plan later [during the patient's stay] to update the goals," she says. "So the care plan was great on admission, but it didn't capture the sense of where we were going, and goal achievement is critical to patient progress and discharge."

Hosta, along with Deborah Quimby, RN, BSN, CRRN, senior director of admissions and case management, believed that there must be a better way to not only promote patients' present status, but also create another mechanism for improving hand-off communication among staff caring for patients.

Anatomy of the form

Although everyone at Youville worked from the same initial interdisciplinary care form, the plans of care often varied by discipline after the initial plan of care was created. As a result, nursing and rehab may have thought that they were working toward the same goal for a patient, but their plans of care may not have matched.

The result of that disconnect decreased the quality of patient information being passed from caregiver to caregiver, and it could have affected length of stay, although the latter won't be known until the form has been implemented longer. Youville piloted the form for a few months on a complex medical unit before it went hospital-wide.

"We'll be interested in length of stay going down, but also in continuity of care going up," Hosta says. "Communication and collaboration among caregivers, that's why we want it to work. Everyone benefits if we can get everyone talking about the same goals."

The form was developed by highlighting the key areas of the initial interdisciplinary care plan and it is uniform for all disciplines, so everyone now is on the same page, Hosta says.

The right-hand column on both pages of the form, labeled "Status of goals," is one of the most important features. It allows staff to update the progress of each goal established in the initial plan of care as appropriate to their discipline area.

Another important feature is the "Target discharge date" section toward the bottom of the form's second page. "The case manager can discuss that with the patient and give [him or her] a time frame," Hosta says.

If the team doesn't believe that discharge is appropriate by the date indicated, then the date gets reevaluated. Case managers review all plans of care with patients and families.

Using the form

Youville is a long-term acute-care hospital, so all patients are discussed once per week on every unit, although another type of facility may choose to do so more often, Hosta says.

Youville's average daily census is 140, or about 22–26 patients per unit, and every unit has a regularly scheduled conference one day per week.

All disciplines get together for a team conference, coordinated by the unit case manager. The 60–90-minute conference is attended by a physician, a nurse, therapists, a dietitian, a social worker, pastoral care, and others who report on patients and give their updates on patients' plans of care.

"The benefit of all disciplines coming together is [that] we know what everyone's goals are, [so] we can all work toward the same goals," Hosta says. "If we're all on the same page, we may get patients discharged in a more timely fashion."

Youville's average length of stay is 26 days. "This form really gives anybody caring for the patient that day a true update on what's going on," she says.

Hosta's advice for a facility looking to adapt the form and the practice of using it is to pull out the key areas/goals from the initial plan of care and adopt the weekly meetings. "These meetings provide a means of sharing pertinent information among caregivers."

Nurses are given an opportunity to fill out the form prior to the meetings. Hosta says the benefit of including the nurses in the process is that they know the patients best, so they can feel empowered in the patient-care process and don't view it as "just another meeting."

Another benefit of using the form is keeping a paper trail to complement any verbal hand-offs that occur—especially when employing part-time staff—that is readily available and current, reflecting the patient's present status.

Hosta is hopeful that the form, along with other methods of hand-off communication used at Youville, will be vehicles to enhance collaboration and promote more optimal patient-care outcomes.

Source: **Briefings on JCAHO** June 2006, HCPro, Inc.

Case Study #5: Application of JCAHO's tracer methodology to plans of care

When the JCAHO surveyor arrives on the patient unit, he or she will request the record of a particular patient. These patients may have been selected before the surveyors began unit visits, or they may ask the unit leader to identify records of a particular type-patient.

For example, the surveyor may ask the leader to identify all patients on the unit for more than 24 hours that have a particular diagnosis, or have had certain procedures performed. They are usually interested in identifying patients that are complex in nature and have received care in more than one setting.

After the patients are identified as requested by the surveyor, he or she will ask to review a particular patient's record. It is preferable that the caregiving team for this type of patient be present for the review. If this is not possible, individual members of the team should be able to assemble, if requested by the surveyor. At least one staff nurse will need to join the surveyor in record review.

The surveyor will probably begin the review process by viewing the physician's history and physical (H&P) and initial assessment completed by the registered nurse (RN). If the assessment completed by the RN indicates the need for other disciplines to become involved in the care of the patient, the surveyor will review the assessments completed by these other individuals.

The patient plan of care will be reviewed and discussed. Staff will be asked to discuss the process they use to share assessment findings, if more than nursing has completed an assessment. The problem list will be reviewed.

The surveyor may choose to discuss problems they identify from the assessment findings but have not been identified by staff. They may discuss problems identified by staff for which there is no obvious data source. They are looking for problem identification to be appropriate to the patient. In other words, they are looking for the assessment findings to be used.

Since the records reviewed are of complex patients frequently receiving care in more than one location, the list of identified problems may be long. They will look for prioritization of the problems and ask staff to discuss the process they use for this. They will discuss how problems identified after admission are added to the problem list and how the problems are reprioritized during the patient's admission.

The plan of care will be reviewed to determine if goals are identified at all. If they are, they will be reviewed to determine whether they are measurable. The surveyor will ask staff to discuss the process for evaluating the patient's progress to the identified goals.

Discussion about the process used to revise the patient's plan of care also will be likely to occur. The surveyor will ask staff to discuss any patient problems identified but not addressed during the admission. If the patient is scheduled for discharge, the surveyor will probably inquire as to post-discharge plans to address the problems, that could include handing the problem off to someone else.

The patient's plan of care will be reviewed by the surveyor during the entire discussion. If the plan has not changed in any way since admission, the surveyor will probe deeper for evidence that care was delivered according to the plan. It is unlikely that patients do not change significantly during their stay in the hospital. The plan should change accordingly.

Source: *Interdisciplinary Patient Care: Building Teams and Improving Patient Outcomes,* 2004. HCPro, Inc.

Case Study #6: Tracer for interdisciplinary care

The surveyor asks to review the record of Mr. John Smith. He was admitted to the hospital via the emergency department (ED), where he presented a week ago with increasing shortness of breath.

His admitting diagnosis was heart failure. He was brought in from home by emergency medical services. He was transferred from the medical intensive care unit (MICU) to your unit (telemetry) two days ago. While in the MICU, he underwent a cardiac catheterization with sedation.

The surveyor will begin the tracer by focusing on the care the patient has received while in the telemetry unit. Care prior to the transfer from the MICU will be reviewed after the telemetry unit, and care in the ED will follow this.

The surveyor will also visit the cardiac catherization lab, either before or after the visit to the ED. In each of these settings, the surveyor will review the record and discuss the care of a patient with the same profile as the tracer patient, or as close a match to the tracer patient's profile as possible.

Although completed prior to the patient being transferred to your unit, the H&P and initial nursing assessment are reviewed. From the H&P, the surveyor learns that Mr. Smith was admitted for heart failure. His history indicates he suffered his first myocardial infarction (MI) about three years ago, and another six months ago.

His cardiac catheterization following the last MI indicated an ejection fraction of only 35%. He has been using home oxygen for the past six months, following his last MI. He was in his usual state of health until about two weeks ago, when he started to retain fluid. He has been following a low-fat, low-sodium diet, but has gained 12 pounds in the last week. He has 3+ pitting edema of the lower extremities and he has rales in both lungs, but no wheezing.

The findings from the initial nursing assessment provide the following additional information:

- The patient was very short of breath on admission, even finding it difficult to answer all the questions without tiring.

- His home meds include a variety of cardiac drugs, a diuretic, a baby aspirin, multivitamins, and glucosamine chondroitin for osteoarthritis.

- He has progressed from two-pillow orthopnea to sleeping in his recliner the last several nights. His gait is unsteady as a consequence of the edema.

- He is unable to carry out his usual routine at home, due to his increasing shortness of breath. He now needs assistance to complete his morning hygiene.

- For the past six years, he and a small group of friends have met each morning for breakfast and a discussion of the day's news and events. He has been unable to join his friends the last two weeks. He reports no pain on admission, just weakness and fatigue.

- He lives at home with his 74-year-old wife. He is a retired music teacher in the public school system in town. His wife is retired from the local bank. She is in poor health, having suffered a stroke about five years ago. Although medically fragile, they assist each other in completing their personal tasks.

- They live in a two-story house, with all the bedrooms on the second level. A full flight of stairs must be climbed to reach them.

- Their children all live in other states. They live in a neighborhood where most of the residents have aged together, so they share common interests. A bond exists between them, and they assist one another with driving, shopping, and cooking. This social network has become a surrogate family for many of its members, as it is for the Smiths.

The screening assessments indicate the need for assessment by physical therapy (PT) and occupational therapy (OT), so referrals are sent to both disciplines, following discussion with the patient's physician. Respiratory therapy staff is asked to manage supplement oxygen administration, titrating to maintain the patient's oxygenation above 96%. Discharge planning is asked to evaluate post-discharge arrangements with the patient and his wife.

The surveyor will probably review:

1. The patient's medical plan of care (progress notes and orders).

2. Medication and treatment orders will be discussed with an eye toward the JCAHO's National Patient Safety Goals (NPSG) around telephone orders.

3. The medication management standards will be discussed at length. This includes things like range orders, blanket orders, illegibility and abbreviations used in orders, review of the medication orders by pharmacy prior to administration by nursing, and a host of other issues.

The interdisciplinary plan of care developed since the patient transferred to the telemetry unit will be reviewed and discussed. The most glaring difficulty with many plans is that they are unchanged since admission, regardless of where the patient is in his or her stay.

The problem list for Mr. Smith has changed since admission. The problems identified on admission were:

- Fatigue and weakness
- Need for assistance with activities of daily living (ADL)
- Fall risk
- Unsteady gait
- Inability to carry out usual leisure activities

The screening assessment for rehabilitation indicated the need for an assessment by PT and OT. He also needed discharge planning staff to assess the home environment for the possibility of needed changes to accommodate the patient returning home after this admission. Social service was needed to assess the home situation to ensure the wife remains safe while the patient is hospitalized.

The current problems being addressed by the team are:

- The need for home care to begin visiting the patient to supervise medication administration
- Safe use of the hospital bed and walker the patient now requires

The discharge planner identified the need for home care when he addressed the home environment and talked to the patient and his wife. The discharge planner will also arrange for delivery and setup of the hospital bed.

Pain in the patient's joints has developed since admission and has also been added to the problem list and plan of care. This is being managed by nursing and OT. The patient is now able to manage his own ADL, and muscle strengthening exercises from PT have enabled him to walk with the walker and no additional assistance. Because his gait improved, he is no longer at risk for a fall.

The surveyor will probably ask staff to describe the process they use to develop and revise the patient's plan of care. In this hospital, they explain that the clinical team meets each morning for 30 minutes to review patients' progress, as well as to share findings (problems identified) from any assessment or reassessment they have completed since the team last met.

If this is a new patient to the entire team, or a patient who has since had an initial assessment by any member of the team, the problem list is developed or revised by the full team involved in completing assessments and identifying problems. Team members only need to be present for the meeting if they are involved in the care of a patient. Plans of care are revised, with input from the clinical team actually involved with a particular patient.

Source: *Interdisciplinary Patient Care: Building Teams and Improving Patient Outcomes*, 2004, HCPro, Inc.

Case Study #7: Developing interdisciplinary plans of care

All patients must have an assessment completed by an RN within 24 hours of admission to determine the patient's need for nursing care.

Screening assessments are also completed as part of this initial assessment process, and determine the patient's need for in-depth assessments by nutrition, rehabilitation (PT/OT/speech language pathology), and discharge planning staff. Patients are also screened for the possible presence of abuse or neglect, with referral to the appropriate discipline/agency for an in-depth assessment should signs suggest this to be present.

It is expected that patients will have a plan of care developed to address any identified needs, after this initial assessment and any subsequent reassessments. When only one discipline completes an assessment, this discipline is the only one involved in developing and implementing the patient plan of care.

For all patients admitted, this will always be nursing, so the initial patient plan of care reflects problems identified by nursing. Often, nursing is the only discipline other than the medical staff that is involved in the care of the patient.

For some patients, this continues throughout their entire stay, but for other patients, additional disciplines are asked to become involved in the care of the patient. This request is made by direct physician order, medical staff-approved protocol, or as a result of the screening assessments completed by the RN at the time of the initial assessment by nursing.

When nonnursing disciplines complete assessments, they often identify additional patient problems. It is expected that there will be a mechanism by which these additional disciplines' assessment and reassessment findings will be shared, so the list of patient problems reflects the results of assessments by all disciplines involved in the care of the patient.

It is important to remember that not all assessments lead to identification of patient problems.

Some patients only require care that is of a routine nature. This care can be provided entirely through the use of protocols/standards of care or practice guidelines, or whatever else you may choose to call them. These are established care or practice requirements. Even patients with identi-fied individual problems often have a part of their care provided through the use of protocols.

Think of these protocols as the operating system in your computer. You don't see it, but it is always operating. These protocols are "routine care"—getting an IV, needing help with personal hygiene, or using a vent—that any patient can expect to receive.

Of course, an existing protocol/standard/guideline must be already present for this to be applicable.

In keeping with the computer analogy, think of the individualized plan of care coming into play akin to when a warning box pops up on your computer screen. That warning box appears on your screen because something in your operating system has said, "Here is something that you need to pay atten-tion to." Whatever that is for this patient, needs to be added to the individualized plan of care.

Some assessments, most often those related to "false-positive" screening assessments, indicate no problem at all. Other assessments may indicate the presence of a problem that is inappropriate to begin addressing at the time it is identified. Other assessments reveal problems, such as weight loss for obesity, which the patient may be uninterested in pursuing.

The analogy for these situations is one many of you are already familiar with. It is the situation when one physician asks another physician to see the patient and offer additions to the medical plan of care, if needed.

In some situations, the consulting physician completes the assessment of the patient and identifies no problems other than those already identified, or has no additional thoughts on patient management. In this case, the consult note usually ends with a statement such as, "Thank you for this interesting consult. I have nothing to add to the patient's plan of care at this time. Call me if anything changes, and I will be glad to see the patient again."

The same possibility exists after an assessment by a nonnursing discipline. Assessment findings would be documented but no problem would be identified, or a problem would be identified but there was no interest from the patient in addressing it. Hence no involvement occurs with the patient plan, unless something changes and another assessment is requested, indicating a problem, or the patient changes his or her mind regarding the addressing of a problem.

Documentation

Nursing should maintain responsibility and accountability for coordinating and integrating the interdisciplinary plan of care.

The interdisciplinary plan of care should be maintained in a place mutually agreed on by the clinical team so that all disciplines can document their evaluations of the patient's progress toward achieving his or her goals. If computerized documentation is utilized, all disciplines need access to each other's documentation at all times. Findings available to only one discipline, and plans maintained by disciplines in isolation of each other, defeat the intent of an interdisciplinary process of care delivery.

The interdisciplinary plan of care should be a working document, used by all members of the clinical team to record identification and resolution of patient problems. It must accompany the patient throughout hospitalization.

Members of the team may change as the patient progresses through the continuum of care, but the interdisciplinary plan of care shall accompany the patient throughout the continuum and shall be used by all disciplines to guide the delivery of appropriate care to the patient, exchange information, to hand off care, and document progress toward goal attainment.

Problem identification

Assessments are completed to determine whether patient problems exist. When only nursing staff have completed assessments and identified patient problems, this list will reflect problems identified by only this discipline. In this case, nursing alone will prioritize the identified problems and develop a plan of care to address those needing immediate attention.

But many patients have assessments completed by more than one discipline. As a result, problems may be identified in addition to those identified by nursing. Because of this, there must be a way to share assessment findings from the various disciplines having completed assessments, so that the complete list of patient problems can be developed.

Only then can decisions be made as to which problems have the highest priority. What had been the most pressing problems, before additional ones were identified, may be less critical as the list expands. This list will usually change over the course of a patient's hospital stay, as new problems are identified and others are resolved or controlled. The problem list may be an actual thing or just a concept, reflected in the plan of care current at any point in time.

The following decisions need to be made by the clinical team as to how identified problems are assigned a priority status:

- Will this be done by the RN alone, or will all those disciplines having identified problems have a voice in this prioritization?

- Will the team identifying problems actually vote on this prioritization and assign a priority number to the problems, or will this be done in concept only?

- Will prioritization occur each time the problem list is reviewed and/or revised?

Resolved problems

Problems shall be eliminated from the plan of care as they are resolved (i.e., when the patient meets his or her goals) or when it is clear that the problems cannot be resolved during admission, in which case there is a plan formed to hand off the problem to another caregiver in the continuum of care (assuming continuation is needed).

For example, a resolved problem might be the attainment of the patient's goal to sit in a chair for 15 minutes and hold his grandchild on his lap without having to use supplemental oxygen.

Also consider that situations might occur in which the definitive goal is not met, but progress has been made and the team (or nursing, if they are the only discipline involved in the care of the patient) determines the problem to be controlled (i.e., as met as it can be).

For example, in the previous scenario, perhaps the patient could only sit for eight minutes without the use of supplemental oxygen because of severe respiratory compromise unresponsive to medical intervention. The goal of sitting for 15 minutes was not attained, but this goal might be unrealistic for this patient. So even though the underlying problem was not resolved and the goal was not met, it could be determined by the team that eight minutes is as much progress as the patient can make. This would eliminate the problem from the plan.

Problem statements

Everyone on the care team should consider the following principles when assigning problem statements:

1. Problem statements need to be patient focused.
2. Problem statements must be clear and mutually understood by all disciplines.

1. Problem statements need to be patient focused.

A patient's problem or need statements must be patient focused. Members of the clinical team often incorrectly make reference to things such as, "the rehab plan of care" and "the respiratory plan of care" or "the nursing problems" and "the social worker problems." We need to remember that these are the patient's problems. We are the disciplines that bring the expertise that helps address those problems.

Examples of patient-focused problem statements include the following:

- "No money to buy medications"
- "Does not understand how to change dressing"
- "Unable to get out of bed without two people assisting"

2. Problem statements must be clear and mutually understood by all disciplines.

The problem statements need to be written (or electronically entered), communicated, and developed in words that are basic, understandable terms that do not resemble any particular discipline.

The problem statements have to look like your patient. If they do not, those problem statements begin to look like the particular discipline that authored them. Suddenly, it has become that discipline's problem and, perhaps, other disciplines cannot even understand what is being communicated in the problem statements.

In addition to being patient focused, the examples I gave previously are written in a language that is easily understood by all the team members.

Examples of phrases found in problem statements that may not be mutually understood by the team include the following:

- "Alteration in fluid volume deficit"
- "Alteration in respiratory status"
- "Ineffective coping"

Every discipline believes it knows how to state the patient problem, but often they don't. This dilemma is rooted in our educational models. As a product of the nursing sphere, I know we were taught to assess the patient and identify all possible problems that could befall this patient from now until eternity, and we were taught how to do it in our own language. The same holds true for other disciplines.

What we weren't taught was how to do this together. As a consequence, we learned to state "nursing problems," "respiratory problems," and "nutrition problems," rather than patient problems. Patient problems flow from the assessment and simplify statements of patient deficit or patient response to something.

Prioritizing problems

Once those problem statements have been clearly established, each needs to be given a priority status.

For example, at initial assessment, you have identified six problems with the patient. Many times you cannot begin to address all the problems you have identified, either because time does not permit it or some things are more pressing than others. You must then determine some sort of pecking order; the JCAHO standards talk about "prioritizing" the problems.

When only nursing is involved in the care of the patient, this prioritization is done by the RN—alone or with other nurses.

Now imagine that after your initial assessment other disciplines complete assessments and identify four additional problems. You cannot possibly work with the patient on 10 different things at the same time.

Decisions about prioritizing the identified problems should include the other disciplines that have also identified problems. Otherwise, their contributions become secondary to nursing and the process is leaning toward a nursing process, rather than being an interdisciplinary one.

It's up to each individual organization to decide how it wants to prioritize. You can accomplish this any way you would like. Here are three ideas or models for decision-making and prioritization:

1. **Use nominal group voting.** Gather members of the clinical staff that have identified patient problems and present them with the problem statements. Ask a team member to place the problems in priority order then ask the other team members to vote as to whether they agree. You can do this one problem at a time or all problems at once. You might decide in advance that a simple majority will win, thus prioritization is done by vote. Whichever problem rates the majority of hands being raised becomes a priority. Remember, even if there are only a few patient problems, prioritization is still supposed to occur.

2. **Adapt an existing, well-known model from some other discipline.** One example that seems to have some applicability for use in prioritizing patient problems or needs is Maslow's Hierarchy of Needs. The actual model, as we know it, is a developmental model and has never been assessed for validity or reliability when applied as I am suggesting it be used. However, as is the case with Maslow, your team can think about patient problems or needs for care falling into groups, with first-level problems or needs requiring attention before subsequent levels can be addressed. Part of the design process would need to include decisions about how many groups/levels you include in your model, if you use this process.

If you do employ Maslow's theory, your model might look like this:

- Basic survival problems, such as inability to maintain spontaneous respirations, would form the bottom level of the hierarchy, and these would take precedence over other problems.

- The second tier might include problems around pain, no food intake, or skin breakdown.

- The next level might include problems such as no safe place to go at discharge, no one to help with care after discharge, and inadequate money to purchase medical supplies.

- The next level might include problems related to the patient not understanding how to do something, such as change a dressing or take medications correctly.

If you use this approach, remember there are no absolutes about how many levels to include in the model or what problems fall into the different levels. Some may decide there are only two levels in the model; others may decide there are three or six. It is really up to the group to decide.

3. **Establish that nursing always decides.** In this model, the RN prioritizes patient problems, regardless of the discipline that identifies it. This may be efficient, but it weakens the interdisciplinary nature of the process.

An example of problem prioritization might look like this:

Problem statements:
- Pain
- No money to buy medications
- Stage-two skin breakdown
- No food intake for last four days
- Lives in boarding house infested with rats
- Thick secretions
- Unable to cough up on his own
- Needs help changing dressing on his left buttock

Using the approach of grouping problems into a rough approximation of Maslow's Hierarchy of Needs, your results might look like this:

- Thick secretions at the first level of problems
- Pain, no food intake, and skin breakdown at the next level of priority
- His living situation on the next level
- His need for help in dressing change on the last priority level

You may group the problems differently. There are no absolutes. What matters is that there is a process for the prioritization. You may have decided on another way to prioritize patient problems.

If it works, keep it. If not, you might consider one of the ways I just described.

The design is, again, up to your organization, but prioritization is key, and you must build into the design of that process a provision for reprioritizing patient problems. Priorities should change over time, just as the identified problems change over time. Your patient's highest priority or need right now might look entirely different tomorrow. Your process has to reflect that.

Some settings review the problem list and reprioritize the problems at least once every 24 hours.

The problems can be listed on the left. The next column is where the problems can be initially prioritized. This will be done by the nurse, because that is the only person involved initially. Numbers would be used to prioritize the problems in this sample, but letters or other indicators could be used. Whoever makes the initial priority determination or any revision would add his or her initials.

It is important to remember that any problem identified but not addressed during the patient's admission must still be documented, along with the rationale for why the problem wasn't addressed. In no way does this negate the assessment findings that generated the problem's identification. It is simply a recognition by the JCAHO that sometimes problems or needs are identified that, for a variety of reasons, cannot be addressed during the patient's stay.

Goal identification

Your interdisciplinary process also needs to include a method for identifying patient goals for all the problems or needs you are addressing. Everyone on the care team should consider the following principles when designing your interdisciplinary process for goal identification.

1. Patient goals need to be patient focused.
2. Patient goals need to be clear and mutually understood by all disciplines.
3. Time frames for goals need to be built for change.
4. The goals need to be measurable (i.e., objective) and attainable (i.e., realistic).

1. Patient goals need to be patient focused.
Much like the problem statements, the goal(s) identified need to be patient focused, not discipline-focused. Remember, this is the patient's plan of care. The patient needs to buy into the goal just like

he or she needs to validate your understanding of the problem. If they have no interest in the thing you think is good for them, it is not their goal—that is, the patient needs to be in agreement that the identified goal is, in fact, a goal with which they would be satisfied.

2. Patient goals need to be clear and mutually understood by all disciplines.
As with the problem statements, the goals need to be written in a common language.

3. The time frames need to be built for change.
Goals need to be written with a time frame that will allow for evaluation of the goal and a change in the plan of care.

Change is likely, and it will continue the patient's advancement toward the ultimate goal, which is whatever the patient wants it to be. If you set all goals to be evaluated at patient discharge—and the patient didn't meet the goals you set— it is too late to change the plan. The goal(s) needs to be written in a way that forces evaluation of progress toward it before patient discharge.

I call these incremental goals; others may call them short-term goals. Think of the goal at discharge as the definitive goal, with incremental goals used to advance the patient toward the ultimate goal(s). They can be used to keep the patient on target or to reverse direction early, if needed. If you look earlier at patient progress toward the goal, you can take incremental steps to change the interventions to get the patient back on track. That is why you want some of those goals set in short time frames. The more critical the goal is to the patient, the shorter the time frame.

When setting time frames for your patient goals, your guiding principle should be: "What does this patient need me or us to do for the next [blank] period of time?" Short-term goals can be set for two hours, four hours, a shift, or some other time frame.

4. The goals need to be measurable (i.e., objective) and attainable (i.e., realistic).
Goals need to be measurable and attainable, and relate to an identified patient problem or need. A goal has to be something that you can see, measure, or feel. It has to be real.

An example of a measurable goal would be:
"The patient will eat at least 75% of the food brought from the dietary department during the next 48 hours."

An unmeasurable goal would be:

"The patient will maintain adequate nutritional intake."

What is "adequate nutritional intake"? It depends on the patient and the person doing the evaluation. That is why the problem(s) and goal(s) need to be derived directly from the assessment. You cannot do this in the abstract.

Most disciplines do not know how to set measurable patient goals. They know how to state generalized wishes. Some clinical disciplines do set distinct, measurable goals, but that is not most people's expertise. That is not what we were taught to do and, like the problem statements, we struggle to define a measurable and realistic goal. It does have to be realistic. If your patient cannot possibly gain two pounds a week, for whatever reason, then do not set that goal.

Unmet goals require a change in the plan

After completing their assessments, all disciplines need to be actively involved in identifying and prioritizing the patient's problems and establishing measurable goals. Also, the participating disciplines need to periodically evaluate the goal(s) in which they are involved. Any unmet goal requires a change in the plan. Any met goal requires consideration of a change in the plan. Therefore, it is evaluation of patient progress to the goal that drives the revision of the plan.

Interventions

The patient's progress toward achieving his or her goals and resolving his or her problems needs to be evaluated on a frequency identified in the goal, with interim assessments done at whatever frequency your organization decides is appropriate. This frequency may be different for different disciplines.

Patient response to the particular intervention(s) needs to be evaluated after the intervention, but evaluation of progress toward the goal should occur with a different frequency. Both of these evaluations should be documented. It is the organization's decision where these evaluations are documented, but it must be evident when reviewing the plan of care. Changes to the goal, intervention, or both, will be made as applicable to the patient.

Revisions to the plan of care shall be made whenever staff identify new problems, when the patient meets a goal or resolves a problem, when the patient does not meet a goal, or when goal(s) and/or intervention(s) are revised.

Each organization has to decide how this will actually happen, just as it must decide how the initial plan is developed. Many options are available for this. One is for members of the clinical team to meet together on some predetermined frequency (e.g., every day, twice a week, and so on) to develop interdisciplinary plans of care, evaluate the patient's progress towards his or her goals, and make collaborative changes to the plan of care. Each organization must find the process that works for it. What works in one place will not necessarily work in another.

An important distinction that every member of your interdisciplinary care team must be made aware of is the need to evaluate the patient's response to interventions, as opposed to the need to evaluate the patient's progress to goal.

There is an expectation in the JCAHO standards now and in the future that patients' response to interventions, whatever they may be, must be evaluated because you need confirmation that what you are doing is working the way it was intended.

This way, if your intervention is not working enough, too much, or not at all, you can change the intervention. It is through the interventions that the goal is or is not achieved.

Interventions need to be documented in such a way that a response is recorded each time. Many organizations choose to document patient responses in the patient progress note section of the record. Other sections of the medical record already exist that may also be used to document patient response.

For example, your medication administration record could be used to document a patient's response to medication. If you give a diuretic such as Lasix, you would measure urinary output, and this can be documented on the output sheet.

It all depends on the way you set up your process. As long as patient response is documented after interventions, it does not matter where you record responses.

Source: *Interdisciplinary Patient Care: Building Teams and Improving Outcomes*, 2004, HCPro, Inc.

Patient and family education

About this facility

Saint Mary's Regional Medical Center, Russellville, AK

- 170 licensed beds
- Key service areas: women's and children's, cardiac cath, inpatient rehab, orthopedics, sleep study, wound care, cancer, diagnostic imagery, skilled nursing, MSICU, emergency, home health
- Last JCAHO survey: June 6, 2006

Patient and family education

No prescription is more valuable than knowledge.
—C. Everett Koop, M.D.

Introduction

As healthcare costs such as deductibles and out-of-pocket expenses continue to rise, admission to the hospital can put an incredible financial burden on patients and families. Our goal at St. Mary's Medical Center is to minimize hospitalizations by helping patients establish and maintain control of their chronic illnesses.

The value of education should not be underestimated as a method to reduce the number of readmissions for the management of minor or chronic illness symptoms. Education provides the patient with self confidence to successfully address symptoms with the techniques taught by the nurse. Additionally, education builds self esteem, which empowers the patient to manage certain aspects of his or her chronic illness at home. For example the diabetic patient is taught how to manage his or her diabetes when they have a "sick" day and experience vomiting and/or diarrhea. With a strong foundation of knowledge, the patient can manage these symptoms at home and not have to be hospitalized unless the symptoms worsen or become unmanageable in the home setting.

The Education Record utilized at Saint Mary's is a dynamic document. It is always evolving as accreditation standards change in the healthcare industry. The last major overhaul of the form took place in 2003 by a multidisciplinary team consisting of nursing, respiratory therapy, case management, social work, and physical and occupational therapy. During this overhaul, legends were added and each discipline was asked to refine the form's wording to be more specific, objective, and measurable. A copy of our current form can be found at the end of this chapter.

The Joint Commission on Accreditation of Healthcare Organizations has surveyed Saint Mary's using an earlier version of this form and complimented the facility for the comprehensiveness of the Education Record.

This chapter will discuss the components of St. Mary's patient and family education tool as well as the facility's overall philosophy concerning patient education.

Education: A systematic process

At Saint Mary's we believe education must follow a systematic process that can always be replicated. This process begins immediately, and the initial teaching begins at the time of admission with orientation to the room to improve patient safety.

St. Mary's educational process consists of the following:

1. An accurate **assessment** that identifies readiness or barriers to learning. The educational assessment conducted at the time of patient's admission will change as the patient begins to respond to medical treatment, which will reduce some of the barriers that may have existed at the time of admission but are resolving, allowing the patient to be more receptive to education.

2. A **plan** concerning how education will be integrated into the patient's treatment.

3. The **implementation** of the educational plan and ongoing adaptation to the patient's clinical situation.

4. An **evaluation** of the educational deliverables to ensure learning has occurred. This gives the healthcare provider the opportunity to re-teach important elements that the patient may have misunderstood.

Assessment

The educational assessment is started at the time of the initial nursing assessment, which the RN completes within eight hours of the patient's admission to the hospital's nursing unit.

This nursing assessment and the establishment of the patient's plan of care cannot be delegated to any other healthcare provider, and many states require that an RN perform the nursing assessment.

The educational assessment is designed to uncover the status of the patient's readiness to learn, his or her preferred method of learning, and his or her barriers to learning, which will ultimately develop a baseline for education. A lack of health literacy—a concept that denotes not only the patient's ability to read but also to comprehend and act on medical instructions—can influence health outcomes.

Establishing the patient's, or in the case of a child, the parent's preferred method of learning is imperative. As adults, we all have varied ways that we best process information and store it in our memory bank. Some persons can simply hear an explanation and be able to comprehend and apply what is taught, while others may have to actually perform a task before it is learned. Because of this factor, educational materials should be prepared in a variety of mediums to meet the patient's learning style.

Nursing staff must also briefly reassess this educational assessment prior to educating the patient for the first time. The nurse should ensure that the education is

Timely—Educate or reinforce education at every available opportunity. Look for "teachable moments."

Individualized—Focus on the patient's specific needs, and adjust the teaching method as needed.

Proportional—Match the amount of education to the needs of the patient.

Specific—Tell the patient/family exactly what they need to know.

Plan of care for the patient's education

Education is an essential part of the patient's treatment plan of care, and must be planned. At Saint Mary's, all of our nursing documents are on a computerized system (EZ ID). Documents are printed in real time at the nurse's station with the appropriate patient identification preprinted. All admission nursing documents, including the Multidisciplinary Patient and Family Education/

Teaching Record, are printed at the time of the patient's admission and are begun at the time of admission.

If you refer to the educational tool included in this book, you will see the educational record begins with a brief assessment of the patient's barriers to learning. The nurse will need to address these barriers immediately so he or she can capitalize on those "teachable moments," or moments when the patient is free from distractions such as nausea and pain and is able to concentrate on the education the nurse is providing.

Barriers to learning can include the following:

Physical

Physical barriers may need to be addressed with the assistance of other healthcare disciplines. For example, if the patient has experienced a cerebral vascular accident and has dominant-hand weakness, the nurse should consult the physical therapist or occupational therapist to discuss if the patient may need assistive devices or if he or she needs to work on cognitive functions to improve his or her ability to learn.

Cognitive

Research has shown that 45% of people aged 65 years and older read at about the fifth-grade level or less. Another 30% read between the fifth- and eighth-grade levels. For older adults, choose easy-to-read materials written in plain language, familiar words, and short sentences.

Emotional

Emotion plays an important role in education. Patients or families who have received a poor prognosis or troublesome healthcare information may be preoccupied and unable to participate in education. Be sensitive to this and provide written materials for the patient to take home if active teaching is not a possibility during admission.

Pain

Experiencing pain may block the patient's ability to learn. Administration of medications for pain relief may also sedate the patient or make it difficult to concentrate on education.

Language

The most obvious barrier to learning is if the patient does not speak English. If the nurse and patient do not speak the same language, the nurse must plan for the utilization of the hospital's translator service.

Cultural

Based on the location of your facility and the population it serves, cultural and religious practices may be a factor to consider when providing education. Too numerous to mention here and because they are very specific to each patient, such practices are also to be considered in planning healthcare delivery.

Motivation

A patient or family member must engage in education in order for it have an effect. Attempting to teach a topic that is perceived as unimportant or not applicable is a waste of energy and time. Obtain the patient's interest by pointing out why the education will be helpful to his or her health-care situation. Don't be reluctant to talk candidly with the patient about what is preventing him/her from participating in the process. Only then will you know if it is appropriate to proceed. To prepare for the educational session, it is important for the nurse to discuss once again with the patient which learning methods he or she prefers. Based on how he or she is feeling, his or her preferred method may change with each educational session or topic. As part of this assessment the nurse must address all the domains of learning including cognitive, affective, and psychomotor.

Cognitive domain

The cognitive domain covers memory, recognition, understanding, and application. Patients master each level of cognition in order of difficulty. For education to be effective, the nurse must first assess the cognitive abilities of the patient so that the nurse's expectations and plan are directed toward the correct level. Teaching above or below the patient's level of understanding may lead to frustration and discouragement. For example, a nurse may find that a patient with Alzheimer's disease may not be capable in this domain due to memory loss, decreased recognition, understanding, and application. The nurse must then adapt the plan to fit the patient's ability.

Affective domain

The affective domain describes changes in attitude and the development of values. In affective learning, nurses consider and attempt to influence what the patient and family think, value, and feel. Since the values and attitudes of the nurse may differ from those of his or her patients, it is important for the nurse to listen carefully to the patient and family and try to detect feelings that may influence their learning. It is difficult to change deep-seated qualities such as values, attitude, beliefs, and interests. To make such changes, patients need support and encouragement from those around them to reinforce new behaviors. For example, in some rural areas, patients and their families believe that certain herbs, such as garlic, can control high blood pressure. Some patients believe that if they take the garlic, they will not need blood pressure medication. It is the nurse's responsibility to educate the patient and his or her family about the importance of taking medication for high blood pressure.

Psychomotor domain

This domain includes the performance of skills that require some degree of coordination. Patients are often taught a variety of psychomotor skills, such as giving injections, measuring blood glucose, and changing dressings.

One example of learning within the psychomotor domain is the diabetic patient who must learn how to perform finger-stick blood-sugar tests. To prepare for this educational session, the nurse first must obtain a glucose meter. These meters come with written instructions and a kit with all the necessary equipment to perform the blood glucose monitoring.

To teach the patient the nurse would first review the written directions with the patient, then have the patient put batteries in the meter, calibrate the meter, and understand the acceptable blood glucose ranges. These tasks have to be understood by the patient prior to attempting the next step of actually "pricking" his or her finger using the appropriate technique, putting a drop of blood on the strip, and inserting the strip into the glucose meter. In this example, the nurse has used reading, listening to the nurse's instructions, doing, and viewing to teach this patient.

Sometimes, a combination of learning methods will help the patient understand the information more clearly. For these psychomotor skills, St. Mary's nurses have been creative in their education delivery and provide the patients with written material along with a supporting videotape, a demonstration, and a return demonstration to illustrate the task that the patient must eventually perform on his or her own. The nurses document their teaching methods by using the teaching method codes (at the top of the education tool), to assist other nurses who will be providing an additional education session so they can utilize and build upon those methods.

Implementing the patient's educational plan

After assessing and planning a patient's education, the nurse can now implement the educational plan and teach the patient and family. There are certain educational guidelines that should be followed for all patients:

- Present information in a logical and integrated manner, from simple, foundational concepts to more complex topics. These should be the building blocks of the education to be presented.

- Reduce difficult or confusing concepts to their component parts and show the patient how to reassemble the components one at a time.

- Pace the information to match the ability of the patient and leave adequate time for the patient to absorb the information. The nurse must remember this is new information, which will lay the foundation for a patient's compliance with managing his or her illness or disease process.

- Maintain continuity for the patient by repeatedly emphasizing essential points. Patients learn better when they are actively involved in the learning process.

The nurse should examine the patient's Education/Teaching Record and review any prior teaching to build on the patient's informational and educational foundation. The patient's education record should reflect previous education and mention if topics need to be reviewed. If there are gaps in the patient's understanding then a review of previously taught information must take place before going on to more advanced education.

To educate patients effectively, the nurse needs to understand the basic sequence of instruction. When the nurse understands these nine steps, he or she can systematically implement education that will maximize the instruction. These nine steps are

1. **Gaining attention**—Before learning can take place, the nurse must gain the patient's attention. One way to accomplish this is by convincing the patient that the information about to be presented is important and beneficial to him or her.

2. **Informing the patient of the instruction's objectives**—Before teaching begins, the major goals and objectives of instruction should be outlined so that the patient develops expectations about what

he or she is supposed to learn. For example, a newly diagnosed diabetic will be sent home on insulin injections. The objective is to effectively treat the diabetes diagnosis and prevent life-threatening symptoms of hyperglycemia and/or hypoglycemia.

3. **Stimulating recall of prior learning**—Before teaching begins, the nurse should ask the patient to recall previous knowledge related to the topic. This assists the patient in linking new knowledge with prior knowledge. For example, if a nurse is teaching subcutaneous injections for the administration of insulin and the patient does not understand how to draw up the correct dose, the nurse should not proceed with teaching about the injection until the patient is able to competently draw up the correct dose of insulin.

4. **Presenting the stimulus**—The essential elements of a topic should be presented in as clear, organized, and simple manner as possible. The nurse should present information in a way that is congruent with the patient's strengths, needs, and limitations.

5. **Providing learning guidance**—For long-lasting behavioral changes to occur, the patient must store information in his or her long-term memory. With guidance from the nurse, the patient can transform general information that has been presented into meaningful information that the patient can recall.

6. **Eliciting performance**—Patients should be encouraged to demonstrate what they have learned. Nurses should expect the patient will make mistakes during the educational process. The nurse can help correct his or her errors and improve skills.

7. **Providing feedback**—Nurses should provide feedback to patients to assist them in improving their knowledge and skills. Patients can then modify their thinking patterns and behaviors based on this feedback.

8. **Assessing performance**—Nurses should be evaluating performance of the knowledge and skills taught. By using the education record, the nurse can assess performance using the response/evaluation legend at the top right-hand corner of the tool.

9. **Enhancing retention and transfer of knowledge**—Once the patient has attained a baseline level of knowledge and skills, nurses should assist patients in applying this information to new situations.

By using these instructional principles, nurses can help patients maximize the learning experience. If steps of this process are omitted, superficial and fragmented learning may occur.

Evaluating the patient's educational plan

The final phase of the educational process used at Saint Mary's is evaluation. Evaluation must take place to ensure that learning has occurred, however this step often receives little attention. Without examining the results during and at the end of the educational sessions, nurses cannot make accurate conclusions about the efficiency and effectiveness of the teaching provided. Fortunately, due to new accreditation and federal regulations, legislation, and increasing interest from healthcare consumers, there is a heightened interest in the evaluation and measurement of patient outcomes.

The nurse can use a variety of approaches, methods, and tools to evaluate educational and behavioral changes. These include questionnaires, surveys, skills demonstration, testing, subjective patient feedback, and direct observation of improvements in the patient's performance and recall of the instruction. Qualitative or quantitative strategies may also be used depending on the nature of the expected outcome, such as changes in knowledge, skills, abilities, attitudes, behavior, health status, and quality of life.[1]

At Saint Mary's we use skills demonstration by the patient and a review of the patient's understanding through behavioral changes to evaluate if patient education was effective. If a nurse finds the education was not successful, he or she documents the patient's lack of knowledge in the Response/Evaluation section of the form with a "NR" or "needs review." This would indicate the patient is not able to apply psychomotor or affective changes.

Approaches to evaluating education effects will vary, depending on the situation. For example, when considering the patient's ability to perform a psychomotor skill such as a dressing change, viewing the actual performance of the skill is the most appropriate means of evaluation.

It is important to evaluate both short- and long-term health and behavioral effects of education.

For example, a short-term evaluation of whether or not a patient can perform insulin injections requires minimal energy, expense, or time. Skill mastery can be determined within a matter of minutes. If the short-term objective is not met, the nurse determines why and identifies possible solutions so that successful learning can occur. If the short-term objective is met, the nurse can then focus on the long-term evaluation designed to assess the lasting effects of the education—in this case, that the patient will perform ongoing daily injections independently during hospitalization and when discharged home.

The ultimate goal of education is to help patients make lasting behavioral changes that will improve their overall health status and prevent future hospitalizations.

Note

1   P. Hawe, D. Degeling, J. Hall, *Evaluating Health Promotion: A health worker's guide.* (Philadelphia: MacLennan & Petty, 1990).

Bibliography

Hawe, P., D. Degeling, J. Hall. *Evaluating Health Promotion: A health worker's guide.* Philadelphia: MacLennan & Petty, 1990.

Martin, K.S., N.J. Scheet. *The Omaha System: Application for community health nursing.* Philadelphia: Saunders, 1992.

Stanhop, M., J. Lancaster. *Community Health Nursing, Promoting Health of Aggregates, Families, and Individuals.* St. Louis: Mosby, 1996.

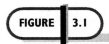

St. Mary's Multidisciplinary Education/Teaching Record

FIGURE 3.1

Learning Assessment / Barriers	Preferred Learning Method	Teaching Method Codes	Response / Evaluation
☐ No Barriers / Ready ☐ Pain / Discomfort ☐ Physical Barrier ☐ Language Barrier ☐ Cognitive Barrier ☐ Cultural / Religious ☐ Emotional Barrier ☐ Poor Motivation **(Check all that apply)**	☐ - Reading ☐ - Listening ☐ - Doing ☐ - Viewing	**A** = Audiovisual **E** = Explanation **H** = Handout **G** = Group Class **D** = Demonstration	**AK** = Applies Knowledge **SI** = States / Identifies **RD** = Returns Demonstration **NL** = No Learning **NR** = Needs Review

Education Needs ☒	Information Relayed / Procedure Instructed	Date	Person(s) Instructed	Teaching Method	Response / Evaluation	Staff Initial & Discipline
☐ Orientation to room / Patient Safety ☐ N/A	Call light, phone, bed control, side rails, temperature control, mealtimes, lab draws, visiting, TV, smoking policy, pt. identification, etc. N/A (cognitively impaired, no family)					
☐ Hygiene/ Grooming ☐ N/A	Bathing/oral care, hair and nail care, toileting N/A (self care or cognitively impaired)					
☐ Med Use ☐ N/A	Describe use of new medications (list) to include action, dosage, precautions, side effects, administration schedule, food-drug/drug-drug interactions, herbal/dietary supplements. ☐ Medication brochure given and explained.					
☐ Dietary ☐ N/A	Modified diet, tube feedings, or other nutrition interventions. N/A (no interventions)					
☐ Assistive Devices/ Equipment ☐ N/A	Walker, cane, crutches, wheelchair (safe and efficient use) N/A (no assistive devices)					
☐ Physical Therapy (PT) ☐ N/A	Rehabilitation techniques, exercises. N/A (no PT involvement)					
☐ Skin Care ☐ N/A	Incision, Wound, or Pressure N/A (no interventions)					
Fall Prevention	Fall Risk and Precautions / Pamphlet given Fall Preventions (all patients) ☐ High-Risk Fall Precautions	FALL PREVENTIONS INITIATED ON ALL PATIENTS				
☐ Pain Management ☐ N/A	Symptom management for pain, nausea, dyspnea, use of pain scale, goal setting ☐ Pain management brochure given and explained. N/A (no pain)					
☐ Discharge Planning/ Case Mgmt Assess & Educate for: ☐ N/A	☐ Community Resources ☐ DME ☐ Home Environment ☐ Discharge Disposition ☐ No Needs Identified ☐ Other:					
☐ Respiratory Therapy (RT) ☐ N/A	Treatment/therapy, oxygen administration, equipment, disease management, etc. N/A (No RT interventions)					
Plan of Care	☐ Plan of Care reviewed and explained					

Init	Signature	Init	Signature	Init	Signature

FAX OR COPY TO NEXT LEVEL OF CARE

Multidisciplinary Patient and Family Education/Teaching Record

«PatientNumber»

ACCT#«PatientNumber» MR#«MedicalRecordNumber»

«AdmitDate»

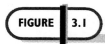 **St. Mary's Multidisciplinary Education/Teaching Record (cont.)**

Learning Assessment / Barriers	Preferred Learning Method	Teaching Method Codes	Response / Evaluation
☐ No Barriers / Ready ☐ Pain / Discomfort	☐ - Reading	A = Audiovisual	AK = Applies Knowledge
☐ Physical Barrier ☐ Language Barrier	☐ - Listening	E = Explanation	SI = States / Identifies
☐ Cognitive Barrier ☐ Cultural / Religious	☐ - Doing	H = Handout	RD = Returns Demonstration
☐ Emotional Barrier ☐ Poor Motivation	☐ - Viewing	G = Group Class	NL = No Learning
(Check all that apply)		D = Demonstration	NR = Needs Review

Education Needs ☒	Information Relayed / Procedure Instructed	Date	Person(s) Instructed	Teaching Method	Response / Evaluation	Staff Initial & Discipline

Init	Signature	Init	Signature	Init	Signature

FAX OR COPY TO NEXT LEVEL OF CARE

Multidisciplinary Patient and Family Education/Teaching Record

«PatientNumber»
ACCT#«PatientNumber» MR#«MedicalRecordNumber»
«AdmitDate»

Nursing Assessment, Plan of Care, and Patient Education: The Foundation of Patient Care

Case Study #8 Measuring the effectiveness of patient education materials

Do patients actually read this stuff?

Do patients actually read the patient education material that your hospital provides to them? How effective is it?

The patient-safety task force at Wadsworth-Rittman Hospital in Wadsworth, OH, asked these same questions last year and decided to get some answers. They surveyed a sample of patients to learn whether the hospital's patient-safety brochure actually helped patients understand their rights, responsibilities, treatments, medications, and other important matters.

The results surprised them: Only 21% of patients said they actually read the information physicians and nurses gave them upon admission.

This was clearly a patient-safety issue, since physicians rely on the material to reiterate information that patients need to know about their care.

"Physicians now spend so little time with their patients that communication has been very sadly eroded. Written information helps prevent miscommunication," says **Jeff Morris, MD**, vice president of medical affairs, and chairperson of the hospital's patient-safety task force.

Problem: According to feedback from patients, the brochure was too long. Patients suggested that it be "broken up" with pictures and graphics. Some also expressed difficulty understanding some of

the language in it, says **Beth Winter, MA**, a task force member and the hospital's public relations director.

Possible solution #1: Hypothesizing that more patients would read the pamphlet if it was simply packaged in a more appealing format, the task force changed the design, added pictures, and rechristened it a "Guest Guide" brochure. The effort, however, was met with a tepid response. A second survey of patients revealed that readership had increased by only two percentage points.

Debra Molnar, coordinator of the hospital's Vintage Club—a loose assembly of current and former patients who are at least 55 years old—began meeting with some of the club's 6,300 members to learn more about their perceptions of the material.

She learned that patients continued to find it "intimidating" and difficult to read. To learn why, she combed research literature and found that the average adult is most comfortable reading at a sixth-grade reading level. The hospital's brochure, meanwhile, had been written at a high school/college-age reading level.

Possible solution #2: The task force is once again rewriting the brochure. This time, they'll write it at a sixth-grade reading level to make sure it's easy to understand and fun to read.

Once the brochures are complete and have been in circulation for six months, the task force will survey another sample of patients to find out whether the changes will increase readership.

This is the best approach, according to John Juergens, RPh, PhD, a researcher who specializes in the literacy level of patient education material. Using small words and illustrations with your text will make it more "user friendly" and understandable, he says.

"A lot of people might be embarrassed to say that they don't understand something. Patients don't want to appear ignorant or less than sophisticated," says Juergens, associate professor of pharmacy administration at the University of Mississippi School of Pharmacy in Oxford.

Tip: As a precaution, nurses and physicians should always ask patients whether they have any questions about written material they have received and should "gently quiz" patients on the content by asking them to paraphrase it in their own words.
"You have to do it in a way that isn't threatening or uncomfortable for the patient," says Juergens.

Tip: Build this kind of questioning into your routine encounters with patients, especially elderly patients.

"Older patients grew up being taught not to question anything that they receive from the doctor or pharmacist," he says.

Such gentle quizzing with patients might have helped Wadsworth-Rittman Hospital's patient-safety committee realize sooner that their patient education material was written at a college level.

"We were overestimating the reading level of the average person who comes into the hospital," says Morris. "Even though we'd rewritten it, it still wasn't at a level that the average patient could comprehend."

About 48% of Americans struggle with low health literacy, resulting in poor health outcomes and costing the healthcare system up to $73 billion in added expenses every year, according to the American Medical Association, which worked under a two-year, $1.5 million grant from Pfizer to identify ways in which providers can help patients become more health literate.

Leadership support is key

Leadership at Wadsworth-Rittman Hospital has been very supportive of the task force's efforts, notes Morris. That's because the task force includes not only Morris, but also members of the hospital's board of directors.

"This kind of involvement is important because if the board sees a patient-safety initiative as important, it sends a very strong message to the medical staff of the importance of providing a safe environment for patients," he says.

Source: HCPro, *Just Ask* Series, February 2004

Case Study #9: Beware of boring brochures

Patients do judge books by their covers

Make sure that the cover of your patient-safety brochure isn't cold and intimidating. That's the advice the patient-safety committee at Gundersen Lutheran Medical Center, a network of hospitals and ambulatory facilities based in La Crosse, WI, received from its 14-member patient-safety advisory council.

The committee asked council members to read two of the patient-safety brochures that the hospital system routinely provides to patients upon admission, and to comment on each brochure's readability.

Consider their suggestions and feedback to help you evaluate your own materials:

Re-examine the cover

The committee recently put an aerial photograph on the cover of its patient-safety brochure that showed all of the structural improvements underway at its massive hospital.

However, the advisory council, which includes former patients and members of the community, told them the picture made the hospital look ominous.

"We were really surprised by this," says **Kim Weber-Chandler, RN**, patient-safety coordinator.

"We were really proud of the improvements that we were making to the building and thought it would be an impressive picture, but they thought it looked really cold and impersonal."

Instead, the advisory council suggested that each cover depict a nurse taking care of a patient.

The patient-safety committee promptly took their advice and changed the cover.

Don't assume you both speak the same language

The advisory council also commented on some of the language in the brochure, and suggested that they replace certain words that, although common among healthcare providers, were not as easily understood by patients.

For example, patients suggested that they replace the word "adverse" with "bad."

"It still amazes us how much we take for granted about what people will understand," says Weber-Chandler.

"Things that we assume are commonly understood in the medical profession are [often] not understood by our patients."

Don't mail brochures to patients
Elderly patients receive so much healthcare-related junk mail that they might set it aside and never read it.

Place brochures within easy reach of family and other visitors
Place the brochures in the cafeteria and on a table in the patient's room. This will encourage family members and loved ones who visit the patient to pick the brochure up and read it.

Source: HCPro, *Just Ask* Series, February 2004

Case Study #10: Patient education: Keep it simple

Simplified patient education is more effective

Effective patient education can lead to greater patient satisfaction, fewer post-surgery visits to the emergency room, and fewer return visits to the ambulatory center. But is your current patient information policy working to that end? There's always room for improvement, say healthcare professionals.

The Joint Commission on Accrediation of Healthcare Organizations' (JCAHO) **PC.6.30** standard requires that the patient receive education and training specific to the patient's abilities appropriate to the care, treatment, and services provided by the organization.

Identify barriers in your facility

Be aware of the obstacles your patients face. For example, some patients may have literacy, language, sight, or hearing disabilities.

Deb Phillips, RN, MSN, a patient-education coordinator at Reading (PA) Hospital and an affiliated, off-site ambulatory surgery center in Pennsylvania, receives medical information at a 12th-grade reading level. Her job is to bring it to a sixth-grade reading ability because most people read between a fourth- and sixth-grade level.

Tricks she uses to make this adjustment include

- scoring reading ease and grade level of the created material (see
  http://csep.psyc.memphis.edu/cohmetrix/readabilityresearch.htm for instructions)

- keeping the length of sentences to 15 words

- using words with no more than two syllables

- making use of 25% of each page's white space

- staying away from symbols such as brackets

How do your patients learn?

One of the top ways to figure out how to educate patients best is to ask them what works, says Phillips.

"As part of our admission database, we ask patients what the best way they learn is—by visualizing, hearing, or doing," Phillips says.

Phillips' centers have also effectively used focus groups to learn what works best. "We try the material on people who are close to the specific diagnosis situation," she says. Phillips also reminds her medical peers that patient education might not always sink in right away—what the JCAHO calls the "readiness to learn" (standard **PF.1.7**).

For example, newly diagnosed cancer patients might be in denial and won't want to hear their instructions—and you can't force-feed the information. The problem then becomes, who will pick up the ball after the patients leave?

Ask yourself the right questions

If you are considering updating how your facility delivers patient education, ask yourself the following questions:

- What do you want to teach?
- What do you already have in place?
- What resources do you have?

Make this a team effort, says Phillips. "People tend to get turned off if this is a solo project," she says. "It's too much work for one person." Instead, help your team understand how effective patient information helps the facility's outcomes.

Source: **Briefings on Ambulatory Accreditation,** January 2005, HCPro, Inc.

Case Study #11: Three ways to involve patients in shared decision-making

The Institute of Medicine (IOM) has identified shared decision-making between patients and physicians as one of the healthcare industry's six principal aims of the 21st century.

"A patient-provider partnership is needed to ensure that decisions respect patients' wants, needs, and preferences and that patients have the education and support they require to make decisions and participate in their own care," the IOM wrote in the 2000 report, *Envisioning the National Healthcare Quality Report.*

To this end, ensure that all conversations you have with patients and all of the educational materials you give them help them understand the following four key areas:

1. The risk or seriousness of a patient's disease or condition

2. A patient's preventive or treatment options

3. The risks, benefits, alternatives, and uncertainties of each option

4. The patient's own comfort level with the shared decision-making that he or she engages in with the physician

Researcher **Stacey Sheridan, MD, MPH,** assistant professor of medicine at the University of North Carolina at Chapel Hill, devised the above list. She specializes in patient-education techniques and offers the following tips to help you achieve the above goals:

Feed information to patients in chunks. Don't expect patients to digest a huge plateful of information at once. Most people have a limited short-term memory that allows them to remember only three to five facts very well, she says.

Help patients absorb and retain important information by supplementing written material with a series of conversations spread out over several visits whenever possible, says Sheridan, who published a study in the January 2004 *American Journal of Preventive Medicine* about how physicians can encourage patients to engage in shared decision-making. The article is titled "Shared Decision-Making About Screening and Chemoprevention: A Suggested Approach from the U.S. Preventive Services Task Force."

Encourage patients to ask questions. Continuously remind patients that you expect them to ask questions and express their concerns.

Research has shown that patients can have better outcomes if they feel that they have a strong say in their care and if they feel that their caregivers listen to them.

Be careful when using numbers. Some patients have a hard time understanding probability concepts that are expressed with numbers.

Make sure patients understand all of the numerical information you provide before they make decisions about their treatment.

Example: Instead of stating that there's a 20% chance the patient will have a bad outcome, tell the patient that 20 out of 100 people are expected to have a bad outcome.

Many people have a hard time understanding percentages, she says.

Source: *Briefings on Patient Safety,* February 2004 HCPro

Putting it all together

Putting it all together

In this book, we have shared the experiences of three nursing leaders who revamped the core documents primarily utilized by nurses in delivering patient care. All of the authors shared the same goal: to develop a tool that would be user friendly, embraced by nurses, and actually utilized. They wanted a tool that when truly integrated into the nurse's day-to-day activities it would be so helpful that the tool's removal would make the nurse wonder how in the world he or she could have possibly functioned all this time without this document.

The three documents represent the natural process of care. Assess the patient to determine individual needs, develop a care plan that will drive consistent care, and provide education to the patient and family. When another caregiver reviews these completed documents, the documents should "tell the story" of the care the patient has received.

Even though we have presented these chapters for nursing, we continue to strive to integrate assessments, care planning, and education with other healthcare professions. Some organizations have been more successful than others. We should not stop here. Perhaps we can stimulate more interest in integrating healthcare if we step into our patients' shoes.

For example if we were to place the physician's history and physical alongside assessments by other disciplines such as nursing, respiratory therapy, physical therapy, occupational therapy, etc., how much duplication in core information would we find? Doesn't that mean that we have asked the patient and family the same questions over and over again? Most likely, the answer is yes. To decrease this inefficient repetition, let's begin to think about the assessment as building blocks of information. Be it a nurse, physician, or another professional, let his or her initial assessment serve as our core data set and seek additional or more detailed information specific to the discipline as supplements. Packaged together, we would have a very detailed picture of the patient that would be more efficient to obtain with less repetitive patient questioning.

Occasionally, we see this building block concept operational in emergency departments. There is one list of medications obtained, one set of vital signs, one history, etc, and all disciplines work from these entries. To do this requires trust in and respect for the other person's skill to accurately and completely collect information.

How will this book's documents stack up with the regulatory agencies?

You will note that there is limited reference to Joint Commission on Accreditation of Healthcare Organizations (JCAHO) standards in the preceding chapters. This is intentional as we believe that doing what is best for the patient will yield regulatory compliance. Yes, it is necessary to know the basic requirements of patient care practices as stated in regulatory publications but consider this: what were the references for writing many of the standards? Of course, they were the principles of the various patient care disciplines.

As a consultant, an impetus for writing this book was continually identifying clients who were struggling with assessment, care planning, or patient education, or all three. In many cases, the root cause was from the organization over-interpreting the standards or attempting to comply with surveyor-specific recommendations, presented as JCAHO requirements, which resulted in the creation of complex processes that were nearly impossible to implement. An overwhelming theme I found was that during patient tracers, healthcare facilities that mastered assessment, care planning, and patient education were far more successful in their mock surveys and in subsequent triennial surveys. Because the method of review by JCAHO is open medical record review, these three documents could either make or break the tracer activity.

With that said, I know that some readers may still be thinking about the required JCAHO components related to these documents. Let's do a brief compare and contrast to set your minds at ease.

Assessment

First and foremost, let's review the definition of assessment as used in this book and in JCAHO's Provision of Care chapter. Assessment is the structured process of obtaining appropriate and necessary information about the patient to assist in planning care, treatment, and services. It is NOT referencing the monitoring or evaluation of a patient that occurs before, during, or after procedures. It is

NOT an evaluation of processes of care that may be conducted by various disciplines. Control your organization's definitions so you do not turn this simple process into a mammoth endeavor and create policies and procedures that exceed 25 pages.

JCAHO's standard PC.2.20 requires a hospital to define the data and information to be gathered during assessment and reassessment. This gives the hospital wide latitude in determining the settings where assessments will be done and what the scope of that assessment should be. Think carefully about this. As we have learned in Chapter One, an assessment collects the necessary information we need to plan the delivery of care, usually over time. If you are an RN working within the radiology department, and your responsibility is primarily to administer medications and monitor the patient's response to invasive procedures, you are concurrently assessing and intervening based on the individual patient's physiological signs and symptoms. You may only be with that patient for a very short period of time. Is a full nursing assessment warranted? You will not be developing a care plan as your care is somewhat pre-determined based on the procedure to be performed and other nursing care is spontaneous in response to the patient's needs. Wouldn't a better use of your time be to educate the patient on the procedure itself, obtain baseline vital signs, and review the patient's history and physical? Perhaps a focused nursing assessment that collects certain information deemed necessary for the planned services could be developed. The fourth element of performance within this standard lists several topics to be included in the assessment and includes a very key phrase, **"as relevant to the care, treatment and services."** Again, permission is granted to define what is appropriate for your organization's settings and disciplines.

PC.2.120 requires the hospital to define the time frame for conducting the initial assessment. Element of performance #3 allows 24 hours to complete the assessment, so do not restrict yourself to time frames that your staff may have difficulty adhering to. I have often seen hospitals that have interpreted the word "conducting" as initiating and therefore define time frames such as "within 15 minutes of arrival to ICU." Be realistic. If the patient arrives in ICU requiring implementation of multiple care items, an actual assessment may not even be initiated for several hours. That is perfectly acceptable as long as your policy allows it and the assessment is actually completed within 24 hours.

PC.2.130 says do what you say you are going to do. Implement your organization's assessment policy and procedure. It is a simple as that.

PC.2.150 addresses patient reassessment. There is only one element of performance: Each patient is reassessed as needed. So why do I find hospitals that have greatly complicated reassessment by adding all kinds of parameters and requirements? If the organization does not live up to its specifications, then you are considered non-compliant. Doesn't the element of performance say it all? **"As needed"** is the key word to safe and appropriate practice in all disciplines.

Care Planning

PC.4.10 leads the care planning standards. Development of a plan for care is individualized and appropriate to patients' needs, strengths, limitations, and goals. The applicable seven elements of performance are:

1. **Individualized** to the patient's needs (just as stated in the standard)
2. Based on the **data from assessments**
6. Patient **needs, goals, time frames, settings,** and services required to meet the needs and goals determine the plan of care
12. **Evaluation** is based on the goals and plan of care
13. Goals are **revised** when necessary
14. Plans are **revised** when necessary
17. Plan includes **strategies to limit** the use of restraints and seclusion

I have highlighted the key words that should be considered in care planning. This is thoroughly covered in the care-planning chapter but worth repeating again because as a consultant, I see staff generating a high-tech, long list of problems and tasks that are driven off a diagnosis and have nothing to do with the patient's individual needs. Further more, care planning is seen as a task to complete a form and the form is never touched again because shift report and physician orders drive the nursing tasks.

Let's change that by focusing on why the patient is in the hospital and what you as a nurse can thoroughly address during the patient's stay. You are not miracle workers. Resist your tendency to list multiple entries of "potential" problems. The fact is, if the patient is in the hospital in today's economic climate, he or she probably has enough "real" problems to address, so be realistic. If you are a relatively new graduate, work with a seasoned colleague to undo what you learned about care planning in your academic setting. The two academic and practical approaches are completely different.

If you are generating a care plan and never looking at it again, why bother? When nurses plan their daily care based only on physician orders, they underestimate our profession's ability to apply critical thinking skills and be a valid part of the patient's team of caregivers. The patient's care plan should be updated frequently and used as the tool for ongoing care, shift report, and to inform other disciplines. Reread Kevin Drew's chapter if you still feel that care planning is laborious and only a paper function. I believe it will motivate you to consider a change in practice.

PC.5.10 simply says that the delivery of care should match what the care plan says.

PC.5.50 focuses on the need for an interdisciplinary, collaborative approach to care planning. Although the rationale indicates that a single care plan is not required, if other disciplines continue to document on separate forms, the nurse, as the primary care giver, needs to review their plans to ensure coordination is happening.

PC.5.60 is the ultimate standard regarding care planning. It wraps up all the requirements into one neat package that supports best practice for the patient. Let's look at the standard by listing the para-phrased elements of performance:

1. Care is **coordinated** through internal resources
2. **External** care is **coordinated**
3. There is a process to share **relevant patient information** to promote continuity of care and services
4. There is a process to resolve **duplication or conflict** of either internal or external sources of care
5. Activities detailed in the plan of care occur in a **time frame** that meets the patient's needs

Regardless of the tools you use, whether they are discipline specific or a common form that focuses on the patient, care is to be timely and coordinated. Do not make this harder than it needs to be. Focus on the basic care that the patient needs for this hospitalization. List the interventions that are working to achieve the established goals. And make this process dynamic—change it as often as necessary to ensure it is a working document.

Pay close attention when defining in what settings care plans are actually needed. Historically, nurses have often generated care plans for surgical services. Ask yourself if this is necessary and adding value to the patient-care process. I believe it fits into the same category as assessment. The patient's stay in the OR is predetermined by the procedure being performed. The patient's care is formulated by the planned procedure and the results of concurrent physiological monitoring. Nursing care is continuous and dynamic in this setting. Planning care is unrealistic; it would be like having a care plan in the emergency department. Use the time you normally put into filling out that piece of paper or screen for "care planning" into providing more hands-on patient care.

Education

PC.6.10 begins by stating that education provided should meet the patient's needs. Here is your opportunity to focus and not feel that you must jam years of education into a relatively short patient stay.

Pay particular attention to the second element of performance: "The assessment of learning needs addresses cultural and religious beliefs, emotional barriers, desire and motivation to learn, physical or cognitive limitations and barriers to communication, as appropriate." During tracers, I often see facilities skip this educational assessment yet multiple entries of education exist. If nurses are not cognizant of their patient's educational barriers and readiness, how will the education be successful? Note the inclusion of these items in the form developed at Saint Mary's Regional Medical Center.

Element of performance #3 lists multiple types of educational topics that should be included for the patient **as appropriate.** Do not miss the "as appropriate" or you will set your expectations too high and try to cover topics not necessary for the specific patient. It is perfectly fine to list the proposed topics on the education form as this prompts staff to assess if this is an appropriate topic for the patient.

PC.6.30 addresses the delivery of education. On Patricia Dolan's form, a column is provided to document if the staff instructed the patient or the family. This is important to ensure that the multiple staff who are educating are including the patient and family members, as warranted.

Content and teaching styles are critical if indeed the patient or family are to recall the education received once the patient is discharged and attempting to continue applying the principles that were taught. Go back to your assessment. Are you capturing the patient's preferred method of learning? Do not proceed without this information. As discussed in the education chapter, we all have a particular way in which we process and retain information. Prepare your materials in several different media to meet different learning needs. Even those patients who state that discussion is the best way they learn may need hardcopy documents to refer to after discharge. Be careful not to impose your learning styles onto patients or families. Be innovative! Consider videos that feature hospital staff, printouts from approved Internet sources, PowerPoint presentations accessed from your hospital's Web site, puppet shows for children, etc.

Tips in developing documentation forms or defining screens for data entry

To further assist you in incorporating these documents in your everyday practice, follow these tips that will set your documentation on the path toward compliance:

- Collect information only if you are going to use it

- Document it once, and only once

- Eliminate the use of narrative notes when information is already documented on forms, flow sheets, etc.

- Maximize the use of charting by exception

- Scale down those busy forms and screens; keep it simple

- In the legend for a form or a dropdown box for data entry, indicate that if a field is not checked, it is not applicable to the patient, or add an N/A checkbox/dropdown field

Your organization's forms, whether hardcopy or electronic, establish the expectations for documentation. They are the record that operationalize your policies and procedures.

Forms that are incomplete may result in your organization being considered non-compliant with your own policies and procedures during external evaluations of your practices. This is why the last bullet point is important.

Remember that these documents should build off one another and be consistent. The assessment should identify the needs, the care plan should document the interventions to meet the needs, and the education should supplement meeting the patient's needs according to his or her treatment and condition. Keep it simple and meaningful. Do not get hung up with multiple sheets of paper or screens that are more burdensome than helpful. As nurses, we can do this, and do it well. I'm counting on you to go forth and spread the word.

Success factors to implementing an interdisciplinary patient care process

Any new process or program that brings about change is going to encounter barriers. In this chapter, we discuss some of the critical success factors that need to occur at your organization before your model of care delivery is to become truly interdisciplinary.

The first barriers that must be overcome are the barriers to change. The design of the process has to incorporate factors for successful management of change, including the following:

Get senior leadership to invest time and energy—Use your leaders to communicate goals, progress toward those goals, and other key messages. Also have those same leaders use employee feedback and input to mold future strategies relating to the process. This demonstrates a commitment to change from the top.

Gather feedback—There should be both formal and informal ways for gathering employee feedback. Feedback gathering needs to occur throughout the change process, as opposed to delaying gathering strategies until after the tools are complete and the process has been rolled out. Your methods for gathering feedback might include:

- anonymous surveys or questionnaires
- education evaluation forms for learners
- follow-up meetings with units
- regularly scheduled mealtime meetings
- posts to an online database

A plan needs to be in place for giving that feedback due diligence and responding to feedback in a timely fashion. Employees need to know their voices are being heard.

Develop a mechanism to track performance—Clearly defined measurements need to be established in the design of any new program or process. Without these measurable performance goals, you will not know if you have actually succeeded in reaching your desired outcome. This is an essential element of the Joint Commission on Accreditation of Heathcare Organizations (JCAHO) performance improvement standards. Hospital leaders are required to consider the hospital's performance goals as they establish or change any services or programs.

Emphasize that the change is here to stay—Let everyone know that the process has no end point. Get them to understand what role the change plays in the organization's vision and emphasize the patient needs that are at the root of this change.

Two levels of critical success factors apply to this change:

1. Factors associated with the design of the process
2. Factors associated with the implementation of the process

The most significant success factor at the design level is getting and sustaining senior leadership support for the change.

Senior leadership support

Individuals cannot undertake something as encompassing as a care delivery model alone, so they must seek approval to launch a design project. If it is the senior leader of the organization, the proposal for the project will probably be presented to the Chief Executive Officer (CEO)/Chief Operating Officer of the facility.

If it is a staff member that has the idea, he or she will probably discuss the idea with an immediate supervisor. This person will need to present the idea of a design project to the person to whom he or she reports, with the proposal ultimately making its way to the Chief Nursing Officer (CNO), then to the CEO. Like any request for organizational support of a project, a proposal will need to be developed.

Organizations are different in terms of how many levels of leadership exist between the staff and the senior leader. Likewise, they are different in how many members of the senior leadership team must approve a project like a change in the patient care delivery model.

Because the work involved in designing the process of interdisciplinary planning and delivery of care will require the organizational resource of staff time, someone at the senior level of the organization must approve the care delivery design project.

This process is not something that can simply bubble up from the grassroots. The idea can come from the staff level, but staff cannot approve the allocation of organizational resources. Senior leadership, whether it is the CEO, vice president of patient care, CNO, or the entire leadership team, needs to be presented with a business plan. They need to know what the goals of the design project are, as well as the benefits, costs, and any additional resources needed for the project.

At South Shore Hospital in South Weymouth, MA, the campaign for senior leadership support started with the hospital's CEO. Going to him for the resources needed to design the process and the resources needed for education and training meant the task force had to make sure he understood the importance of this change, and why it needed to occur. From there, the task force educated the vice presidents. The task force had representation at the vice presidents' division meetings, where the vice presidents met with their leadership—their directors.

When you look at the resources you need to roll out this type of initiative to staff, you need 24-hour, seven-day-a-week coverage. This is a staffing issue that senior leadership needs to understand. For training and education to be executed successfully across the care team, staffing resources need to be allocated and hospital leadership has to commit their participation in the implementation process.

Managers also need to be prudent when looking at their current resources, asking themselves, "What are my internal resources? What are my external resources?"

At South Shore Hospital, Donna Chase, RN, who is director of education and training, had the following resources play crucial roles in rolling out the design team's training and education plan:

Off-shift educators

Two off-shift educators worked a 6 p.m. to 2 a.m. shift. They rounded on the units during the evening and night shifts, educating staff who were ordinarily difficult to reach.

Night, weekend, and holiday supervisors

A group of night, weekend, and holiday supervisors were used as part of the education team for reaching staff who may not be on-site for regularly scheduled information sessions. These leaders were used as double coverage, adding education duties to their administrative purposes.

Information specialist part-timers

Although her primary staff is nursing-based, three part-time information specialist educators were on staff. Usually dedicated to using and teaching software systems to staff, the role of educator was an easy fit.

Chase also looked at nurses who were out on workers' compensation. She sought employees who could not come back to do physical work but could help roll out the process. As a result of this strategy, she received large contributions from a nurse who spent six months on the process before she was ready to come back to her actual job.

These types of resources also may be available in other departments within your organization, as well. Potential trainers and educators may be current full- or part-time staff members who can flex-up their hours, or former staff members who are out on workers' compensation and related issues. Keep in mind that education does not require that you do physical lifting.

Team-building experts

If approved, the first task will probably be to assemble a group of individuals that express an interest in working on the project. Some organizations may choose to appoint individuals to the design team. The individuals will need to be educated about the project, including the characteristics of the interdisciplinary care model. As they are educated, team building must also begin. This is perhaps as critical as the sharing of factual information.

Representatives from various clinical disciplines will be assembled for the design team and might not even know the other people in the group. They likely have no real understanding of each other or how to work as a team. Unless the separate individuals begin to function as a team, the work of designing a process to support the concept of interdisciplinary care will likely stall.

Teams do not develop by themselves. Someone in the organization, perhaps from human resources, who is experienced in helping individuals become a team will be needed early in the project. If no one inside the organization has this skill, someone from outside the organization will need to be found. It would be counterproductive to bring individuals from separate disciplines together and tell them to work as a team to design an interdisciplinary care model, with no assistance in learning how to work together as a true team.

Once the tools have been designed and your interdisciplinary care process is in place, other factors will determine the future success of your process.

Support from all disciplines involved

There are two components to this factor. Earning support from all the disciplines involved means getting all those disciplines represented and included at the design level. You need to have all the right disciplines at the table, and you have to assure that their contributions are reflected in the process.

The second component occurs after the tool and process has been generated with interdisciplinary support and buy-in. The question becomes: How do you ensure that support and buy-in permeates the staff of these various disciplines?

Each component consists of two very different audiences. The first component is likely to be a group of leaders—your directors of the various clinical disciplines, and key medical leaders. The second group is made up of the actual bedside care providers from those disciplines—your rehab therapists, your dietitians, and so on.

An example of how important support is from all disciplines can be found by taking a closer look at your organization's assessment tool. In rehabilitation services, the various therapists, regardless of whether it is occupational, physical, speech, or something else, all like to document in their own sections of the chart. They document care very well and they are comfortable with their documentation.

Yet, an interdisciplinary care process would require that everyone document their care goals for the patient on an interdisciplinary plan of care.

How then does the director of rehabilitation services, who was involved in the development of this process, assure that he or she can sell this to staff, resulting in the organization's goal for a true interdisciplinary care process? This question applies to any director whose discipline is involved in patient care. The director of dietary, spiritual services, occupational therapy, and so on, all need to convey this concept to his or her staff.

One of the strategies that has worked successfully is for these leaders to gather as a management team and discuss methods for communicating the benefits and value of this change to staff. These communications should be unified, so all the disciplines are getting the same message and everyone understands the message is coming from a unified leadership.

If this cannot be done effectively, your process is going to be swimming upstream because the leaders are not the ones doing the documentation—the care providers are.

In addition, compliance challenges tend to emanate from change that is not perceived as value-added. The best way to improve compliance is to have everyone understand the change and, more importantly, understand the value of the change. This involves leaders acknowledging that although this interdisciplinary process is a different way to document, it's a better way to document.

To help ensure his or her participation, each clinical team member needs to understand the benefits and the value of this process. This begins by showing team members the significance of an interdisciplinary plan of care tool, for example' and helping them recognize that now there is one location for any discipline, including the medical staff, to see the key clinical goals for a particular patient.

An individualized interdisciplinary plan of care keeps all of this information in a consistent location, making it much easier for everyone on the team to make sure that there has been appropriate problem prioritization, and that care is on the right track.

Right now, when goals are scattered throughout the medical record, the clinical staff could lose sight of certain ones and cannot effectively prioritize what needs to be done for the patient. How can goals be effectively prioritized if the chart is an inch thick and the goals are scattered throughout? It is almost impossible in that scenario to uncover all of the goals.

It is also important for staff to consider that the average length of stay for a patient is approximately three days. The care team cannot address every patient need in those three days; therefore, the prioritization process is essential. The care team's focus needs to be directed toward the key clinical goals and objectives of the patient. This will also enable it to potentially make a dent in that patient's length of stay, adding more value to this process. This key value drives everyone's goal, which is to get patients out of the hospital as quickly and safely as possible.

If, however, your organization has determined that your existing documentation system (each clinical discipline documenting in a separate section of the medical record) has been extremely successful, then it is important for discipline leaders to explain the value of the new process as it relates to that system.

Each member of that clinical team has to understand the importance of bringing their key goals over to the interdisciplinary plan of care. Although this would result in duplication of documentation, it would be minimal. Staff has to understand that either approach is acceptable, and the value is having that unified, central location for tracking care of the patient and a system that fits your organization.

Physician involvement (starting at the top)

Each organization has a different medical staff model, and it is essential that you understand how best to communicate and encourage the support of your key medical leaders if your interdisciplinary patient care process is to succeed. Having physician representation in the development of the interdisciplinary care-planning process will greatly enhance your ability to help the physicians understand the value of this process.

If no physicians are involved in the development of the interdisciplinary process and you do go back to the physician chiefs and ask for their help, it will be significantly more difficult to get their assistance. It is a given that everybody on your care team appreciates the ability to have input to assure their discipline is appropriately represented in the process. Nobody likes to have a final product handed to them and then be asked for their contributions, physicians included.

Physicians will document their goals in their physician documentation, but what needs to be assured in an interdisciplinary process is that none of the physician's documented goals conflict with the goals identified by the interdisciplinary care team. Having an interdisciplinary plan of care tool available and acknowledged by physicians is a key element in the success or failure of your interdisciplinary care process.

No standard says all the physician's documentation needs to be included in this interdisciplinary plan of care. Some organizations have seen the value in documenting in this method. Some have found it more advantageous to have the physicians documenting their plan and goals in the physician progress notes. Either approach is acceptable. Other approaches are also acceptable, as long as there is a way to identify conflicting goals or outcomes.

In behavioral health and rehab settings, physician involvement is done well, but this has yet to be replicated in the medical/surgical units. Organizations working on this challenge have debated several different techniques for securing physician involvement.

One design team debated putting a box on the plan of care that the physician would be required to mark, as if to say, "I've reviewed the plan of care, and I concur." The difficulty with that was that the physician would have to do that every time the plan of care changed. That could result in an unreasonable amount of busywork for them to do.

Another proposal was to ask the physicians to make a general statement in the progress notes, merely acknowledging that the plan of care was there. This team also talked about adding space for a note at the top of every progress note page where the physician could acknowledge the plan of care. In the end, this facility never found a consensus, and the process failed.

Another plan at another facility had physicians participating in rounds that were done in part to review patients' plans of care and make changes to them then. Another idea was to designate somebody who could actually meet one-on-one with the physician to help facilitate the review of that patient's plan.

Whether your process involves stickers or stamps, notes or rounds, the point is that there are a number of ways to accomplish this. What matters most is that you determine the method that is internally comfortable for your organization's culture.

South Shore Hospital's success in designing and implementing its interdisciplinary patient care process in 2003 hinged on physician leaders' support and their influence on the physicians in their group. In 2000, the task force's medical executive committee was made up of volunteers. At times, the task force's initiatives were met with resistance due to the physicians' other commitments.

Having physician leaders who can sit with the discipline directors of the hospital and plan together is important. In 2003, South Shore had paid chiefs of the primary services at the table, such as chief of surgery, chief of obstetrics, chief of medicine, vice president of medical affairs, chief of pediatrics, and so on. These were employees of the hospital, and therefore more understanding of the task force's objectives.

These physician champions are the hospital leaders that you need to help the physicians understand their role in this interdisciplinary process. The task force met with these physician chiefs every other week, and these physician leaders helped drive some of the work it took to reach their physicians.

Getting the buy-in from those medical staff leaders began by educating them about the benefits and value of the process. Keep in mind that the learning objectives do not change whether you are speaking to these physician champions or the physicians in their groups.

Establishing a common language

An interdisciplinary patient care process will not survive without addressing the different languages used by the various disciplines on the clinical care team.

Each discipline has a language that they have been taught in their education and have enhanced during their clinical practice. Physical therapists tend to speak in "modalities," respiratory therapists provide "treatments," and nursing provides "care." You cannot expect problem statements and/or goals that are written in the language of one particular discipline to be understood by everyone involved in that patient's care. Therefore, those identified problems and goals need to be patient focused and written in such a way that all the disciplines can mutually understand.

It is up to your design team to establish and incorporate a common language between disciplines when it develops the tools used to document care. Use of clear communication and a common language between disciplines will stem from a consistent educational approach to the tools.

The goal is to create a hospital-wide language as it relates to the plan of care, and the best way to ensure that a common language is understood and retained is in a strong educational rollout.

Each discipline may recognize terminology differently, so within the education of the process there needs to be an assurance that everyone understands, for example, what the problem list is, and what it is intended to accomplish. Furthermore, by making sure that consistent terminology is used in dealing with a piece of the medical record such as the problem list, you will assure that all the disciplines are using a common language.

The breakdowns occur and barriers go up when the education does not successfully convey the value of the process. When that happens, people tend to look for reasons or opportunities for the process to fail.

Therefore, assuring that everyone is clear on the benefits of the change will minimize the potential for these barriers. This is true whether we are discussing language barriers, practice barriers, or documentation barriers. Somebody is going to find a way to make it fail. The key is getting everyone to want the change to succeed.

All the care providers across all of your clinical teams also need to have consistent communication practices when it comes to bedside care. This is more difficult to evaluate and assess than documentation, but it is a crucial step toward strengthening interdisciplinary care at your facility.

We know from JCAHO's research around sentinel events that one of the contributing factors in all of those situations was unclear communication. To that end, communication is the focus of one of JCAHO's seven National Patient Safety Goals.

Abbreviations are another example of where communication needs to be mutually understood. It is essential that all caregivers—not just physicians—follow approved abbreviations.

Even if a facility has a comprehensive approved and unapproved abbreviations policy, hospital leadership needs to ensure that every discipline is using only approved abbreviations and the computer-generated medications administration record (MAR) is updated. By failing to eliminate unapproved abbreviations from the MAR, the facility was providing an exception to its own policies and endangering patients. Because nurses use the MAR to give medications to patients, the record becomes an important form of communication.

Trigger questions

On an interdisciplinary assessment tool, communication between disciplines is highlighted in the wording of the trigger questions. Typically, nursing will do the initial assessment and ask those trigger questions, but it is essential that disciplines other than nursing be involved in creating those questions that lead to more specialized assessments.

A problem that some organizations have is that when they are developing key triggers that would necessitate a referral, they do not involve the appropriate discipline in the development of those triggers. Without this involvement, your patient care process may be missing at-risk patients.

This means asking the various disciplines—dietary, respiratory therapy, pastoral care, and so on—to think about the key questions that need to be asked during that initial assessment in the first 24 hours that would trigger them from seeing Patient A rather than Patient B. This is the first prioritization exercise that occurs in the patient care process.

Well-developed interdisciplinary trigger questions will always include some type of algorithm. For an example of a well-developed trigger question, South Shore Hospital's Nursing Initial Assessment says under nutritional status:

"If 3 or more affirmative answers to above questions or if patient is unable to answer, contact Nutritional Services for assessment of nutritional status."

That is a very simple and strong algorithm. It tells the nurse: if this, then do that. Even if a hospital has developed some good questions, a badly worded algorithm can lead to inconsistent care. For example, if the nutrition algorithm above had said:

"If any of these questions are positive, consider contacting nutritional services for assessment of nutritional status."

That is not a strong algorithm. This leaves the decision up to the individual nurse. The nurse is not a nutritionist, so he or she should not have to make an interpretation. This needs to be rewritten to say: if this, then do that.

Although no standard exists for what the algorithm needs to be, it must be definitive if it is to be effective. The wording has to be practical, simple, and understandable by every discipline that uses the tool. Trigger questions must be:

- developed in part by the discipline involved in the question
- attached to a strongly worded algorithm

If not, these trigger questions threaten the consistent, quality care that every organization strives toward.

This can occur in any discipline, but often spiritual triggers are a pain point for organizations designing interdisciplinary patient care tools. For example, an assessment tool will include a trigger such as, "What's your religious affiliation?"

That is not a well-crafted spiritual trigger. It is likely that the pastoral care department was not appropriately represented in the design process.

Just because a person is a member of a particular denomination doesn't necessarily mean that that person wants to see a member of the clergy. A more appropriate trigger might be, "What provides you comfort or support? Are there any religious, cultural, or ethical beliefs that would be important for us to know during your hospitalization?"

After that, the tool might instruct the care provider to then ask, "Would you like to see a member of the clergy?" Even if your first trigger reveals that your patient does have strong religious, cultural, or ethical beliefs, the patient still may not want to see a member of the clergy. All of this needs to be followed by a strong algorithm. If the answer is yes, refer them to pastoral care.

Ensuring the process fits your organization

How do you know if the process you have designed fits your organization? You need to understand that there is only one correct way to design a process for interdisciplinary patient care at your facility.

The only correct way is to design the process that makes the most sense for your organization, patient population, and staff. The process needs to be customized to meet your organization's mission, vision, and values.

Source: *Interdisciplinary Patient Care: Building Teams and Improving Outcomes*, 2004, HCPro, Inc.